ME, MY CELLS, AND I

ME, MY CELLS, AND I

A Survivor's Seriously Funny Guide
to the Science of Cancer

DAVE AMES

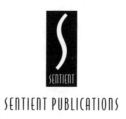

SENTIENT PUBLICATIONS

First Sentient Publications edition 2011
Copyright © 2011 by Dave Ames

A paperback original

Cover design by Kim Johansen, Black Dog Design
Book design by Timm Bryson

Library of Congress Cataloging-in-Publication Data
Ames, Dave.
  Me, my cells, and I : a survivor's seriously funny guide to the science of cancer / Dave
Ames. — Sentient Publications ed.
    p. cm.
  ISBN 978-1-59181-173-2 (pbk.)
  1. Ames, Dave—Health. 2. Prostate—Cancer—Patients—United States—Biography.
3. Prostate—Cancer—Treatment—Anecdotes. I. Title.
  RC280.P7A485 2011
  616.99'4630092—dc23
  [B]
                                    2011017039
Printed in the United States of America

10 9 8 7 6 5 4 3 2 1

SENTIENT PUBLICATIONS
A Limited Liability Company
1113 Spruce Street
Boulder, CO 80302
www.sentientpublications.com

Contents

Introduction

My friends like to tell me I look pretty good for a dead guy. And, no, this isn't one of those vampire books. I'm not really dead; it's just that I'm supposed to be.

Cancer.

Four percent. Fifty percent. Ninety percent. Everything the doctors tell you, from how long you might live to your chances of debilitating side effects, it's all couched in percentages. For me, there was an 80 percent chance I'd be dead in two years, and when I showed up at the Pearly Gates I'd likely be dressed in a diaper.

Saint Peter: "Dude..."

Me: "I know, I know."

Did I mention the diaper would be dirty?

Honestly, I wasn't sure I wanted to live like that. At the time of my diagnosis I was forty-nine years old, and had white stripes between the tan lines on my feet because I'd spent the better part of my life in river sandals. What? Me worry?

I was a fly-fishing guide in Montana. Plenty of fresh air, lots of exercise. I might die of a beer bottle to the forehead after hitting a sour guitar note in a particularly discerning honky-tonk, but then there is no such thing as a particularly discerning honky-tonk. I was going to live forever until that bright October day when the doctor snapped on a thin plastic glove and I wished he had smaller knuckles.

"Bend over," he said.

That was nothing compared to the post-hole digger that came next, and the news just kept getting worse. Over the course of two weeks I went from having never given death a second thought to a 90 percent chance of making it five years to an 80 percent chance I'd check out before I'd paid for my room.

Did I mention how expensive this was all going to be?

I'd managed to side-step these issues for decades because I'd always been pretty healthy. I was like most pretty healthy Americans, a member of the ostrich family, with my head buried in the medical sand. It's like I thought I could avoid cancer by ignoring cancer, and if that isn't the dumbest idea I ever had, it's close.

Having ignored cancer unsuccessfully, I had some catch-up reading to do. Over the next couple of years I would read dozens of books and hundreds of papers. Most of this came after the conventional phase of my treatment, because I just had to believe there was more to it than what I'd been told by the mainstream medical establishment.

For instance, one side effect of my career as a fishing guide was that I knew a lot of prominent doctors. I talked with ten in all, each one smart, a couple near the pinnacle of their respective specialties. But of all those doctors only one even mentioned diet, and if they didn't put much stock in how diet might improve my survival chances, you can imagine how they felt about something like *qigong* (chee-gong).

Snicker, snicker.

"Well...nothing proven...outright quackery...now, back to real medicine."

I'd do it the doctors' way, or one of their ways, because they all recommended different treatments, but the best conventional medicine could offer me was a 20 percent chance I'd see my kids graduate from high school. I'd be a fool not to consider other treatments that might improve my odds, but what would they be?

Doctors, internet, diet books, TV, magazines—we're inundated with conflicting medical advice. Eggs are good for you one month, bad the next. A ballyhooed blood test is diagnostic one year, disregarded the next. A drug is prescribed to millions of people one day, the next it's the subject of a class-action law suit. Conventional medical wisdom changes all the time, so how are we supposed to make educated health decisions?

Cancer sucks. The best you can say for this disease is that you can learn from it, and in my attempt to consolidate contradictory medical advice cancer proved to be the ideal topic to investigate. This was because cancer is a disease of the cell, the indivisible unit of life, and it was at the level of the cell that a clear path finally began to open in the maze of conflicting medical information.

How do our bodies function at a cellular level?

And how does that affect our health decisions?

Those are the questions this book addresses. It's everything I wished I'd known at the time I was diagnosed, but didn't have time to find out. This is the story of what worked for me and it's based on the science, both pro and con, behind a diverse array of conventional and less conventional treatments.

When writing this book, as much as possible, since all experiments are not created equally, I referred to the original research papers. It doesn't matter whether you are investigating the cancer killing power of broccoli or the effect of consciousness on chemicals in the immune system, you can better evaluate the worth of experimental data if you know how those experiments were performed.

In evaluating that data, I stuck to the principle that the simplest answers are most likely to be correct. Like complex lies, convoluted scientific explanations can fall apart at any point along the way. Ask not what your cells can do for you, but rather, what you can do for your cells. Fix your cells and you fix yourself.

That's simple enough, and it was backed by eighty years of compelling research into the interplay of oxygen and cancer. We fight cancer the same way we fight aging, by taking steps to provide our cells with energy, and when our cells have more energy so do we. It was so simple even a fishing guide could understand it, and for the first time in my life health decisions made sense. Unfortunately, just because I knew what I should be doing, that didn't mean I'd do it.

There's a reason they call them habits.

If you're anything like me change doesn't come easily. It helps me if I know not just what to do, but why. If I know how a treatment works I'm more likely to both do it and believe in it. This in turn creates a self-fulfilling prophecy, a feat at which your body excels, because almost any treatment is more likely to work if you believe in it.

I had no idea what I would find when I sought ways to help save my life, and therefore this book reads a bit like a mystery. It's a journey of discovery, and, like any good mystery, it begins with a crime, in this case identity theft.

We Have Met the Enemy and It Is Us

You have, among the over two hundred different types of cells in your body, a roving band of vigilantes called *natural killers*. These immune cells are an important part of your initial response to intruders and, somewhat like border guards, their job is to demand of other cells the proper molecular fragments that identify you as you.

Natural Killer: "Your molecular papers, please."

Invasive Bacteria: "Well, let's see, they were here a minute ago."

Natural Killer: "You are hereby sentenced to death."

Natural killers have the chemical wherewithal to act as judge, jury, and executioner. They can release chemicals that call for backup, they can send out for crews to clean up the remnants after intruders are destroyed. The problem with a cancer cell is that because it once was you, it can sometimes pretend it still is you.

Natural Killer: "Your molecular papers, please."

Cancer Cell: "Hmmm...I do have this expired driver's license."

Natural Killer: "OK, but I'm keeping an eye on you."

Just because that cancer cell passed muster the first time doesn't mean it will the next time. Cancer is a continuum that begins with regular specialized cells in which, in response to environmental toxins or genetics or more likely an accumulation of factors, the DNA responsible for proper cell reproduction becomes corrupted.

The number of cells in a typical human body (100 trillion) is on the scale of the number of grains of sand it would take to stretch between the earth and the sun. With so much to go wrong, it's no surprise that it does. It depends on what we eat and breathe, and it's hard to measure, but estimates of potentially cancerous cellular events per day in any given human start in the millions and go up from there.

This may seem depressing but the good news is actually twofold.

First, and this is huge, by controlling what goes into our bodies we can limit the potentially cancerous cellular events to which we must respond. This decreases the chances of getting cancer in the first place; it also frees up limited resources such as natural killers to attack existing problems, and the more times any given cancer cell is asked to prove its identity the less likely it is to survive.

The second piece of good news is that when the inevitable mutations do arise, we're really, really good at beating them back. Most times immune cells like natural killers don't even get involved. Normal cells have enough self-awareness that when they sense they have become corrupted they commit apoptosis, or self-destruction for the common good.

Normal cells are well prepared to make this sacrifice, but cancer cells over time develop the ability to side-step this altruistic ritual suicide. Cancer cells, in a process very much akin to classic Darwinian evolution, progress through a cascade of genetic changes that build one upon the other to ensure survival and proliferation of the emerging mutant.

For instance, normal cells are subject to chemical signals (both from the brain and neighboring cells) that tell them when to divide and when not to divide. There's an on-switch and there's an off-switch. Cancer messes with both switches by evolving the ability to produce its own growth signals while ignoring signals to stop dividing, and unchecked and self-initiated growth is only the beginning of cancer's tricks.

Normal cells appear preprogrammed to reproduce a maximum of fifty or sixty times over the course of a lifetime. Research shows cancer cells apparently lose this genetic restraint and can theoretically divide ad infinitum. It is a form of immortality that comes with a heavy price because genetic damage compounds with each passing generation. Mutations mount, and the cells become less and less like the cells from which they originally grew. Cells that were once highly differentiated into specialized breast, prostate, or lung cells are now visibly undifferentiated. Irregular blobs replace the ordered shapes typical of normal cells. Internal cellular structures lose definition and function, as the cancer divides and forms a localized tumor.

It's bad, but it's probably not enough to kill you.

In fact, research suggests we wipe out several of these low level infestations over the course of a normal lifetime. These tumors are relatively weak because, up until now, the cancer cells have been surviving largely on the energy produced by the fermentation of sugar, and fermentation is an anaerobic and extremely energy-inefficient process.

Normal cells oxidize sugar, and the oxidation of sugar produces nineteen times more energy than the fermentation of sugar. Normal cells need this extra energy to stay normal, and therefore require an unabated supply of oxygen and nutrients, which is why they generally reside within one hundred microns of a capillary blood vessel.

The ratio of blood to cells, like everything else in your body, exists in a delicate balance. There are just enough blood vessels to supply existing tissue, and cancer cells, as they reproduce, and squeeze between normal cells, are limited by this lack of blood.

A defining point in the progression of a tumor comes when cancer cells, in collaboration with local normal cells, release the chemical signals that result in the growth of new blood vessels. This is called *angiogenesis,* and with a dedicated supply of oxygen and nutrients, the tumor can now grow much more rapidly.

These rapidly reproducing cells can also evolve the capacity to ignore or override molecular signals that instruct normal cells to adhere together. Your organs are your organs because your cells follow chemical messages to stick together in a pattern specific to that organ; when mutants interfere with that chemical code the now untethered cancer cells that grew in one organ can ride the currents of your bodily fluids in search of a new organ to call home.

Mutated cells from one organ colonizing another organ can't be good and it isn't. *Metastasis* is the word that describes the spread of cancer cells beyond the site of the original infestation, and these distant settlements of one kind of tumor cell in another kind of tissue are responsible for 90 percent of cancer deaths.

This was my situation.

Almost certainly.

There are those percentages again.

My cancer was of the prostate, and, at the very least, based on biopsy results, there was a near certainty it had escaped the sheath surrounding this walnut-sized organ. How far it had spread beyond that was anybody's guess, and when a cancer has metastasized you face a whole new set of challenges.

The better you know an enemy, the easier it is to defeat. This is as true of disease as it is of business rivals or warring countries. I was determined to base my decisions on the cellular strengths and weaknesses of cancer as outlined above, and one of the first decisions I had to make was whether or not to have surgery.

About half my doctors recommended surgery as the "gold standard," the rest had other ideas. It was a tough call at first, but since it was metastasis that was most likely to kill me, it seemed the first order of business was to limit metastasis.

It is a strength of cancer that it can grow anywhere it finds nutrients; it is a weakness that it can spread only cell by cell. You can fight metastasis by bolstering the resources your body needs to identify and destroy wandering cancer cells; you can also fight back by doing what you can to limit the numbers of wandering cancer cells in the first place.

There is something to be said for surgery that eliminates every potential wanderer at the source, but my cancer had almost certainly grown into the tissues surrounding the prostate. In removing this organ, the surgeons wouldn't be cutting the tumor out, they'd be cutting through it. This would in turn flood my blood and lymph with cancer cells, any one of which could find nutrients and metastasize into the tumor that would kill me.

Looking at it like this, surgery made no sense.

One decision down, a couple thousand to go.

Hung Like a Castrati

Deciding against surgery meant my conventional treatment would include some form of radiation. Professional opinions varied as to what form that treatment might take, but I opted for a three-pronged approach that most clearly addressed the central premise that my cancer had spread. First, a wide beam of external radiation would be directed in the areas around the main tumor where mutants already likely lurked; second, radioactive seeds would be planted directly into the tumor to attack the core cancer grown fat and strong on a steady diet of testosterone.

Ah, testosterone.

I was going to miss it.

The third prong of my treatment would be drugs that interfered with my body's ability to manufacture and use the hormone testosterone. The reason was that most prostate cells, both normal and mutant, thrive on testosterone, just as most breast cells, both normal and mutant, thrive on estrogen. For someone like me, with a high likelihood that a hormone-driven cancer had spread, hormone deprivation therapy that would starve the cancer of its favorite food source before, during, and after the combined external and internal radiation treatment made utter sense.

No matter where that cancer was in my body it would be affected by testosterone deprivation. Again, I'd be addressing the issue of metastasis head-on. Some wandering cancer cells would be killed outright; many more would be weakened to the point where my immune system could polish them off. With luck the cancer would shrink back to a point where the combined effects of internal and external radiation could nuke every last core mutant, so I drove through a Christmas Eve blizzard to a drug store where I filled the prescription for the drug that would start the process.

"Sir, are you all right?"

My face went white as I stared at the bill.

"Sticker shock," I mumbled.

I was one of an estimated 25 million underinsured Americans. At least I wasn't one of the 50.7 million uninsured. I was paying nearly five hundred dollars a month for catastrophic health insurance with an annual five thousand dollar deductible and coverage limited by a list of exclusionary statements. A new year was coming on; I'd just paid off one deductible and was about to start on another.

Ten grand in deductions, sayonara.

Another five hundred a month in premiums, adios.

There's only one country in the world where that kind of money doesn't buy you full health benefits and I lived in it. Importantly, my policy didn't cover prescription drugs. The twenty pills in the tiny vial came to six hundred and change, money I needed for food and Christmas presents for my kids. I'd be paying for the pills the same way I'd be paying for all kinds of things my insurance didn't cover.

"Charge it," I said, and handed over a credit card.

Credit card debt is both steep and hard to pay off. It's the next best thing to loan sharking, and somewhere, a banker rubbed his hands in glee.

Fourth quarter profits were looking good, very good.

As for me, back home at the round oak table in the kitchen, I stared at a hard white pill half the size of an aspirin. In the bad old days a few decades ago, castration was the only reliable method of lowering male testosterone levels. The pill on the table would have the same effects on my body, but with the distinct advantage that the process didn't involve a knife and was therefore reversible.

In the meantime, I was in for quite a show.

As long as they live, men never quit making the male sex hormone testosterone. Women, on the other hand, at the end of their reproductive years, do quit producing the female sex hormone estrogen, which manifests as the change of life called menopause. Males deprived of testosterone can exhibit, from mood swings to hot flashes, all the same symptoms as women deprived of estrogen. Whatever it was to be female, I was about to experience firsthand.

Most women with whom I shared my fears called it justice.

Finally, they said, a man who can understand.

The Spark of Life

As I sat there staring at that hard white pill I realized I knew quite a bit about the symptoms it might cause, but almost nothing of the why and the how. What would really be going on inside me? And how would that affect the rest of my decisions?

I had no idea.

This preoccupation with effect as opposed to cause is a difficulty every cancer patient in America will face. There's only so much information you can get in a typical fifteen minute doctor/patient office visit. If I wanted the rest of the story I was going to have to find it out myself. So, while I researched that little white pill and radiation therapy, I also researched diet and Chinese medicine, anything that might help.

Questions led to answers that led to more questions that led to more research. Commonalities appeared, and, time and time again, with regard to what at first glance appeared to be vastly disparate treatment disciplines, the element oxygen assumed a starring role on the stages of both cancer and human health in general.

At first, I paid this coincidence no mind.

Oxygen as a cure for cancer?

It was ludicrous, even absurd, yet the more I read the more sense it made. First, oxygen by weight makes up 65 percent of the human body. More than anything else, we are oxygen. Second, oxygen drives the reactions that provide the energy that fuels our cells. If there isn't enough oxygen, there isn't enough energy, and if there isn't enough energy, many problems—including cancer—can result.

The simple logic of it all simply became too powerful to ignore.

The nature of cancer is a function of the nature of the cell. The nature of the cell, in turn, is a function of the properties of water, while the properties of water are a function of the nature of oxygen. The nature of oxygen, in turn, is a function of the properties of electrons, the ultimate source of energy in our bodies, and right now you might be thinking, "Oh-oh."

Right now you might be like Indiana Jones, only it's not snakes you hate.

"Chemistry," you might be saying. "Why did it have to be chemistry?"

In response, I would say, if you're truly interested in finding a path through the swamp of conflicting medical advice, then what is a whole lot worse than learning some chemistry at this point is not learning some chemistry. Plus, maybe someday you'll be asked to be a contestant on the game show "Are you smarter than a fifth grader?"

"...And the fourth grade science question is: 'What do you call electrons in the outside ring of an atom?'

"Hint: they're not called Billy, Bob, Suzie, or Sally."

The answer might be worth fifty thousand dollars to you. The knowledge might be worth even more, because it is at the level of these outer electron rings that so much of the force that drives our lives is played out, and it all begins with water, the medium on which cellular life as we know it is based.

Water is a particularly stable molecule comprised of two hydrogen atoms attached to one oxygen atom. It's about as simple as molecules come, and molecules form because the entire universe, from quasars to cells, in a force as pervasive and irresistible as gravity, is driven by a fundamental tendency toward electric neutrality.

The hydrogen atom is the simplest expression of that electrical truce: one positively charged proton circled by one negatively charged electron, for a net charge of zero. An atom of oxygen, with eight protons and eight electrons, is also electrically neutral, yet neither a single atom of oxygen nor a single atom of hydrogen is electrically content to exist in the universe as we know it.

Electrons orbit protons in energy shells generally depicted as rings. The first ring is considered full (or at capacity) with two electrons; the second ring is considered full with eight circling electrons. Larger atoms can have more than two rings of circling electrons, yet the outer shell is always called the valence shell. This outer ring is where the electrical interplay between atoms that form molecules occurs, and just as the primal forces that drive nature stipulate electric neutrality, the primal forces that drive nature to form molecules also stipulate full valence shells.

If you looked at these first two electron rings like tables in a restaurant, then there would be tables for two and tables for eight. That's it, and no matter how many electrons showed up, every valence table would always be full. This wouldn't be possible except that electrons are the ultimate social butterflies, because they can sit at more than one table at once, through a process called *covalent bonding*.

In a molecule of water, oxygen brings six valence electrons to the table, while two hydrogen atoms bring one electron apiece. That's a total of only eight electrons, but they somehow manage to satisfy the forces of nature by filling two hydrogen tables for two and one oxygen table for eight. Go figure. Covalent bonding is a process that requires a lot of sharing. It probably wouldn't work

THE SPARK OF LIFE

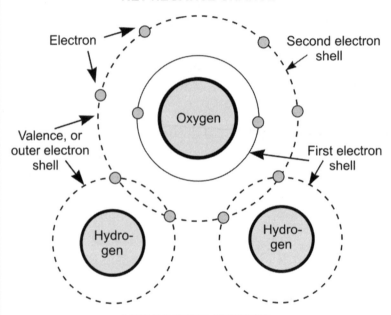

The unequal distribution of electrons in a water molecule creates a particle that is charged like a battery. This molecular spark induces the reactions that power cellular life, and an unimpeded flow of electrons provides energy that leads to good health. If you've been feeling tired lately consider that the food you eat can constipate your electrons as well as your colon, and this is a problem a plunger can't fix. I don't know about you, but it makes me want to go lay down on the couch just thinking about it.

with blocks in a kindergarten, but it does with electrons in the universe, and implies that protons, by nature, are not selfish entities.

Perhaps we all need to get in touch with our inner proton.

In a molecule of water, equal numbers of electrons and protons preserve overall electrical neutrality, but even electrons can't be everywhere at once. Oxygen has a dire thirst (or affinity) for electrons and, in that water molecule, the spinning cloud of shared electrons tends to spend more time around the large oxygen nucleus and less time around the small side-by-side hydrogen nuclei. Since electrons are negatively charged the net result is a polar molecule, where the oxygen end tends to carry a negative charge while the hydrogen end tends to carry a positive charge.

This battery-like polarity provides the spark upon which cellular life is based because nature constantly strives to neutralize that polarity. Opposite charges attract, like charges repel. The polar ends of water molecules will seek out opposite charges in other polar molecules or ions in an attempt to balance the charges. If the difference in polarity is great enough water molecules can surround another polar molecule like a writhing cage, and that polar substance is said to have "dissolved" into the water.

Protein is just such a polarized substance. Protein readily dissolves in water, yet people are largely protein. So, how is it that we can go swimming without becoming one with the lake?

Nearly four billion years ago, when the Earth was fiery and young, riddled with volcanism and bombarded with meteorites, the proteins that would become life in the proto-oceans faced much the same dilemma. In order to form, cells needed a substance to keep all that water at bay, and if you've ever tried to wash a greasy skillet without soap you're already intimate with that material.

Fat.

Fats are nonpolarized molecules that come in many shapes and sizes, yet they share the common nonpolarized characteristic that while they will dissolve in other fats, they do not dissolve in water. Sesame oil mixes with olive oil in the wok, but both oils repel water. The nonpolar nature of fats is a chemical truth upon which cellular life is founded, and, since different cells require different fats, blind devotion to food labeled as "low fat" can be one of the worst things you can do to yourself.

The technical term for fat is *lipid,* and phospholipids are phosphorous-containing fat molecules that line up to form cell membranes. This semipermeable membrane differentiates the chemical environment in the thick liquid (cytoplasm) that fills the cell from the liquid world that surrounds the cell, and is a defining characteristic of life. Similarly, smaller internal membranes within the cell define *organelles* such as the nucleus and mitochondria, and it is in these specialized organelles that the work of life progresses.

So what does that have to do with cancer?

As it turns out, plenty.

Fats are electrical insulators, and the chemical differences between the inside and the outside of a cell are also electrical differences. Positively and negatively charged chemical particles constantly flow through the membranes of your cells as nature tends toward electric neutrality. The same force that drives an atom of oxygen to acquire electrons drives the energetic reactions that fuel life, and any interference with your cells' ability to create and use that energy (say, through the simple lack of the proper fats) means something has to give.

There isn't enough energy to go around. Cells must compensate, and the highly specialized organelles begin to shut down. The fats and proteins that those cells contributed to your life are no longer made, packaged, and delivered. Your DNA is under constant assault from charged particles called *free radicals;* molecular repair crews are standing by only when there is sufficient energy for them to go about their business.

Cells very much resemble factories that receive raw materials and build finished products, and a cell without oxygen is like a factory without power. In a factory, idled and un-maintained machines begin to break down, while once happily employed workers can transform their pink slips into all manner of mischief. Cities with high unemployment are more susceptible to both crime and riots. Order breaks down, and in a cell, over time, idled organelles can lose their function and DNA can be corrupted.

What was once a highly differentiated cell, producing specific material that contributed to the common good that is you, is now a more-or-less undifferentiated blob just trying to survive. If that mutated cell reproduces, cancer has been initiated. There are now two cells where there was once one, and since the flow of oxygen supplying blood remains constant, cancer, as it grows, creates a micro-environment of low oxygen levels that stimulates further mutations.

On the other hand, if your cells have plenty of energy, then so do you.

The Lessons of the Lake

One of my earliest memories is of building sand castles on the beach. The corner turrets stepped up three bucket-tiers high, and olive-drab plastic soldiers stood watch from atop the towers as waves lapped against the shore. It turns out I had the right idea, but it would have taken a lot more than my personal army of miniature soldiers to keep me safe as I ran screaming with delight into Lake Erie.

I've always loved water. I started competitive swimming when I was eight and didn't quit until after college. As for fishing, it's not like I can't remember the first time I fished. It's more like I can't remember a time when I didn't fish, like whatever it was swimming around in the womb with me was fair game, and the fact that I was building sand castles rather than fishing is telling.

In Lake Erie, back then, you never caught anything.

Except, maybe, cancer.

From automobile exhaust to food additives, we live in a civilized world redolent with potential carcinogens. Exposure to these toxins doesn't mean you're going to get cancer, just that there's more of a chance. The greater the exposure, the greater the chance, and the effects of these exposures can take years or even decades to manifest.

Cancer bides its time in a cumulative fashion. For instance, in a river near where I used to swim, liver cancer in brown bullhead catfish increased significantly with age, up to about 44 percent of four-year-old fish, as opposed to control groups, which had no liver cancer. No statistics were reported on five-year-old children, but back then the joke was if you fell in Cleveland's Cuyahoga River you didn't drown, you decayed, so it does make you wonder why the beaches were open in the first place.

This book is about laying a foundation upon which you can base your own health decisions, and part of this is never forgetting that just because the government or a television commercial tells you something is OK to eat, drink, or breathe doesn't mean it is OK. With billions of dollars at stake you don't always get the whole truth.

In fact, a lot of the time you don't get much truth at all.

This is as true now as it was then, and back then Lake Erie was a veritable who's who of potent carcinogens. There were gobs of mercury, and plenty of the particularly nasty polynuclear aromatic hydrocarbons, whose aroma is as familiar as hot asphalt. Other chemicals included industrial PCBs and the insecticide DDT, good examples of how today's technological marvels become tomorrow's lawsuits, because both these substances that were so widely used at the time were subsequently shown to be so toxic that they were completely banned.

The list of toxins in the Lake Erie of my youth goes on and on, and you'd think it would have been enough to kill any lake, but you'd be wrong. Lake Erie died from the same factor that can cause cells to become cancerous: not enough oxygen. In a cell it's called *hypoxia,* in a body of water it's called *anoxia;* either way a lack of oxygen is the linchpin in a chain of cause and effect that ultimately leads to death.

Anoxia in water results from a process called *eutrophication,* and is indicative of processes throughout the natural kingdom in that it shows how too much of one thing can lead to too little of another. In Lake Erie then, and in oceans around the globe now, the "too much" arrives mostly as excess agricultural phosphorus. Phosphorus is a critical limiting factor on plant growth and is therefore concentrated in fertilizers. When more fertilizer is applied to a field than the plants in that field can use, the leftover nutrients leach into the ground water. The phosphorus-rich ground water then percolates into the rivers, which in turn fill the lakes and oceans with too much of a good thing.

Algae bloom so profusely in this nutrient-rich bath that they choke themselves off from the sunlight and die, resulting in a rain of dead algae cells that settle to the bottom of the lake or ocean. This prompts dedicated species of bacteria to then carry out their life's work of decomposition, a process that requires oxygen. So many bacteria feed on so many dead algae that all or nearly all the available oxygen is used up. The animals in the lake then suffocate, beginning with the highest life forms, which need the most oxygen, such as the largest bony fish, and ending with the simplest life forms, which need the least oxygen, such as jellyfish.

In Lake Erie, an intricate system of life forms was rendered less complex because of a progressive lack of oxygen. As normal cells become cancerous, an intricate system of life is rendered less complex because of a progressive lack of oxygen. If you believe you might learn something of the one from the other, a few thoughts surface.

First, I started this chapter thinking Lake Erie would be a good example of how exposure to toxins increases cancer risk factors. But, what I found instead, and would keep finding until it became too obvious to ignore, was that, from cells to oceans, a lack of oxygen was the driving force behind the declining health of a living system.

Second, Lake Erie now supports a world-class steelhead trout fishery. Restoring normal oxygen levels quickly restored complex life, far faster than most experts ever believed possible, and if it worked in the toxic soup that was Lake Erie, it's just one more reason to believe that it can work for our cells.

Third, oxygen levels were restored in Lake Erie by reducing phosphate levels rather than pumping air into the water. This is the difference between treating cause as opposed to effect. It may seem obvious that problems are better solved by addressing cause as opposed to effect, but radiation and chemotherapy very much treat cancer by the equivalent of pumping air into the water.

These conventional treatments treat the symptoms of cancer, but they do nothing to treat the underlying cause. It's true that these treatments may be necessary in the case of advanced tumors, but the idea that these conventional treatments are the only or even the best way to treat cancer is illogical at a cellular level because, as cancer grows, the battleground expands to include the many and varied ways in which cells communicate.

The Hormone Express

Hormones, in general, are chemical messengers that carry instructions from cell to cell. Dozens of hormones constantly carry dozens of messages over both short and long distances. There are messages to go, messages to stop, so many messages it makes a texting teen-age girl, no matter how fast her flying thumbs, look like a slacker.

As an example of just how quickly systems can go awry, consider the following sequence of text messages you might have with a teenage daughter.

Daughter: "Can I go 2 the movies?"

You: "Who with?"

Daughter: "Betsy."

Lately, your daughter has been hanging out with the wrong crowd. You'd really like her to be home by ten, but you've always liked Betsy. All the self-help books say you need to build trust, so you decide to give your daughter the benefit of the doubt.

You: "Be home by midnight?"

Daughter: "LOL"

You notice your daughter has not actually answered your question as the phone blanks dead; on the other end of the line your daughter turns to Bruno.

"You ready to go to the tattoo parlor?" he says.

Cancer subverts your body's messaging process in similar fashion. Cancerous cells send fraudulent messages implying everything is OK when it's not, and cancer sends for the equivalent of more pizza with Bruno. This chemical deception is one of cancer's greatest strengths, and the criminal mastermind that initiates much of this chemical deception is a protein called *Hypoxia-Inducible-Factor.*

There's that oxygen again.

In semi-plain English, this protein is a factor, the production of which is induced by hypoxia, or a lack of oxygen. This protein is a factor because it in turn stimulates the production of several more chemicals, which are released from the cancer cell and into the blood, and very quickly detected by the hypothalamus, a chunk of your animal brain about the size of a sugar cube.

The hypothalamus is a bundle of grouped nerves in charge of maintaining all the delicate balances that result in a healthy you. Data is received from specialized sensory cells about blood chemistry and temperature. The information is processed, and then the constant stream of work orders that maintain your status quo are forwarded to what arguably remains the world's most advanced chemical manufacturing plant, especially when you consider it's only the size of a raisin.

The pituitary gland manufactures and distributes a total of eight hormones on demand into the bloodstream, and these hormones carry chemical directives to other endocrine glands such as the thyroid or the adrenals. Go to the beach and sit in the sun: melanocyte-stimulating hormone signals skin cells to darken through the release of melanin. Get up and go for a swim: thyroid-stimulating hormone increases the rate at which blood glucose is metabolized to provide energy for working muscles. See a black shark fin slicing the waves: adrenocortitrophic hormone pumps up the fight-or-flight response. Go back to the hotel for a little hubba-hubba: follicle-stimulating hormone signals the male sperm to mature, oxytocin signals the uterus to contract during the female orgasm. Cut yourself shaving before dinner: human growth hormone stimulates cellular repair and reproduction.

As you'd expect, when cancer calls for human growth hormone, it's a giant step in the wrong direction. Many lines of cancer research focus on waylaying these chemical messengers en route, yet cancer has proven quite resilient in its ability to slip these messages past the guards. There are too many alternate routes of chemical cascades through which messengers can travel for one drug to block all the back alleys at once.

Again, it's a matter of addressing cause or effect. In this case it's clearly better to provide the cell with enough oxygen to prevent the hypoxia that induces the creation of these chemical factors in the first place, because these chemical messengers, once they've been manufactured, are hard to stop, and harder to destroy.

Most messenger hormones, including human growth hormone, are proteins, and proteins carry messages somewhat like words, if words had to be boiled in acid for several hours before the letters fell apart. The "letters" in proteins are amino acids, and the amino acids are strung together with carbon- and nitrogen-based peptide bonds that cling fiercely to their electrons. Peptide bonds are very strong, and several amino acids linked end-to-end are called, appropriately enough, *peptides,* while a dancing conga line of a hundred or more amino acids in a row is called a *protein.*

There are just over twenty different standard amino acids, most of which your body can make but some of which you have to eat. Each amino acid has very different chemical properties (including shape and degree of polarity), and, when joined together, each amino acid will tug, twist, and pull on every other amino acid in a specific way. Any given chain of amino acids tends to loop and coil back on itself in response to those forces, resulting in a clump of a particular shape. Different sequences of amino acids fold into very different shapes, and it is in those shapes and associated properties that proteins carry their particular messages to other parts of the body.

The eventual destination of that message is the DNA at the center of a cell, yet the polar protein is unable to dissolve and pass through the nonpolar fats that make up a cell membrane. The message can't be delivered directly, so it is instead relayed to proteins imbedded in the cell membranes called *receptors*. This interaction is often compared to inserting a key into a lock, but molecules move, so it's more like mating snakes. At any rate, messengers (or *ligands*) of one shape activate receptors of another shape. This in turn triggers chemical reactions inside the cell that switch genes on and off, which results in the production of still more chemical signals, which in turn control the production of all the various fats and proteins of your life so as to maintain the balances that are you.

If this seems a cumbersome process consider that life did not spring all of an instant into being. Life evolved, over billions of years, from simple to complex, from single-celled to trillion-celled, and these chemical communication processes built one upon the other as the need arose to relay messages over greater cellular distances.

The result is a system of communication that resembles the old Pony Express. Messages are delivered from station to station; at each station the message is relayed forward by a new messenger on a fresh horse. The message might pass through several stations before it is finally delivered, and once the message is delivered, there is always a reply. The reply can be negative or positive, and the dynamic equilibrium provided by the constant exchange of information in these feedback loops maintains the body's chemical concentrations within the limits of life.

Hormones can be built from amino acids but they can also be built from one of the most important fats your body makes, cholesterol. Cholesterol-derived hormones are called *steroids* and, when released into the bloodstream, steroids have the fat-like ability to pass through a cell membrane. It's a more direct way of delivering messages, like the messenger can walk through the door and hand deliver the information instead of leaving a note in the mailbox outside for somebody else to pick up and pass on.

The sex hormones are fat-based steroids. Sex hormones can walk right through the door to deliver their messages, and estrogen feeds some kinds of breast cancer the same way testosterone feeds prostate cancer. If your goal is to deprive breast cells of estrogen or prostate cells of testosterone there are two ways to go about it. You can block the ability of a cell to receive a signal, or you can block the production of the signal, and these are the same two ways all pharmaceuticals work.

Drugs called *antagonists* are engineered to resemble natural ligands, but not quite. Antagonists settle into a receptor and, without triggering a reaction of their own, block the receptor to potential natural ligands. It's like fitting almost the right key into a lock. We've all been there, and it's usually dark and raining. The lock won't open and the wrong key gets stuck, so even when you find the right key you can't use it.

Tamoxifen, the widely used breast cancer drug, is just such an antagonist intended to block the uptake of estrogen receptors. Bicalutamide, the active ingredient in the six hundred dollar vial of little white pills that began my journey into womanhood, was also an antagonist, which blocked the ability of the receptors in my body to accept natural testosterone. This antagonist was administered as a side show to the main event, the injection of another drug, leuprolide acetate, a chemical *agonist.*

An agonist, in the pharmaceutical world, is the opposite of an antagonist. An agonist is engineered to initiate the same reactions as a natural ligand, only more so. The artificial agonist I would be taking had a half-life of three hours, as opposed to a half-life of three or four minutes for the naturally occurring ligand. The chemicals differed in composition by only a single amino acid, yet testosterone-producing reactions that had lasted minutes would now last hours.

In early experiments with these artificial agonists on laboratory rats in the late 1970s researchers expected commensurate increases in overall testosterone levels accompanied by swollen prostate glands; what actually happened was described as a "completely unexpected scientific finding." Testosterone levels initially spiked, as expected, for a few to several days, but then dropped precipitously to post-castration levels. It was as if the rats had no testosterone-producing testicles at all, and subsequent experiments showed that humans were even more sensitive to the effects of these agonists than rats.

There are lessons in this "completely unexpected scientific finding" when it comes to health decisions. First, much of our greatest medical science, from penicillin to X-rays, has happened by accident. Science tends to disregard results it can't prove, yet it is important to remember that this may be only because the right accident has not yet happened. Second, the researchers shouldn't have been so surprised at the unexpected results of this experiment, not if they had studied the lessons of the lake, because this was a classic example of too much of one thing leading to too little of another.

In your body, it happens all the time.

Prolonged stimulation of the circuits in charge of producing testosterone simply fried the circuits, spawning an accidental androgen deprivation industry that did 1.7 billion dollars worth of business in 2008. There are a lot of people out there with a vested interest in messing with your hormones, and I was far from alone as I watched the nurse tapping bubbles from the syringe.

"Bend over," she said.

There are a lot of ways you can get bent over, and I pointed at the needle.

"What's this shot going to cost?" I asked.

The doctor wrinkled his nose as if he'd smelled something distasteful.

"Beats me," he said. "You'd probably have to go to bookkeeping."

I closed my eyes and sighed as the nurse jabbed me in the butt with the agonist that, through the miracle of time-release technology, would deprive my body of its ability to make testosterone for the next several months.

"Bookkeeping," she agreed.

Some costs just can't be measured in dollars and cents. Whatever the price, my pants at my knees, there was no going back now.

A Lesbian Trapped in
a Fisherman's Body

Guys are different than girls, a pervasive singularity that begins with the gonads and ends with the brain. Or maybe it's the other way around. At any rate, the corpus callosum, the main neural pathway connecting the left and right hemispheres of the brain, is proportionately larger in women than men, a connection that has been shown to enhance the ability to speak articulately.

So when it comes to talking, men right off the bat are at a disadvantage. This shortcoming is compounded because the male emotional center is in the right brain and the language specialization center is in the left. Back and forth, back and forth, between hemispheres through an undersized corpus callosum, that's the inefficient mental pathway a man must follow to turn his emotions into words.

By the time a man figures out what to say it's generally not his turn to talk anymore. The woman is way ahead of him since the female brain has emotional centers in both hemispheres of the brain, enabling more direct access to both her feelings and the feelings of others as she puts her emotions into words. Talking between the sexes just isn't a fair contest.

Of course, neither is wrestling, although both can be fun.

The initial differentiation of male and female brains—and therefore what it is to be a boy or a girl—appears to be related to fetal levels of testosterone and estrogen. The female offspring of mother monkeys who were injected with testosterone during pregnancy showed male traits like aggressive play and mounting behavior. Castrated newborn male rats grew up to develop a larger left brain hemisphere, a female trait. Conversely, newborn female rats with their ovaries removed developed larger right brain hemispheres, a male trait.

Certainly, there are no absolutes in the male-female spectrum. Some men talk better than some women and some women wrestle better than some men. Both men and women produce both estrogen and testosterone, although men generally have forty to sixty times the amount of testosterone in their blood as women. Other key differences include the facts that women's levels of estrogen (and other hormones) fluctuate wildly each month as an egg is prepared for potential fertilization, and that women's ovaries cease production of estrogen when eggs are no longer prepared for fertilization at the end of reproductive life.

These are natural (yet not necessarily welcomed) hormonal processes for a woman, but it is in no way natural for men to be deprived of testosterone. Men produce testosterone all their lives. To a certain degree men *are* testosterone. All over my body, cells that for the last fifty years had grown accustomed, even addicted, to a steady supply of testosterone would suddenly be deprived. Any or all of those cells, in any or all of the systems in which they were found, could be affected.

This is one reason drugs have side effects: because the receptors with which a drug interacts are located in cells other than the target tissues. There's really no rhyme or reason to the distribution of any given receptor throughout the body. It's just a function of the haphazard nature of human evolution that tended to re-use chemical components rather than trying to reinvent the wheel each and every time, and this conservation of useful chemicals is seen throughout the plant and animal kingdoms.

A second reason drugs have side effects is because, to continue with the example of the Pony Express, when a single horse arrives at any given relay station, the message can trigger the release of several horses. A king may receive a message that the country is under attack; he in turn sends many message-bearing horses to notify his dukes and earls, who in turn send out still more horses to notify their soldiers. If you interfere with any one of those horses you interfere with all the horses that are to follow.

When you take a drug, the ensuing web of chemical reactions and dead horses is individual, specific, and impossible to predict. Some people get one side effect, some another. For instance, one out of every three or four men deprived of testosterone report symptoms that include general pain along with both constipation and diarrhea (you can see how that would be painful). The most commonly reported side effect, in over half the men, is hot flashes, and I was part of the half that got them.

Wow.

Having gone through it, here's my advice to husbands. If your wife is having hot flashes, go buy her some flowers. She needs them.

A hot flash is aptly named; out of the blue, at totally random times, in the middle of a bite or the end of a sentence, for no discernible reason, you begin to perspire. Your skin flushes, your heart pounds, your breath catches. From moments to minutes you're uncomfortably hot, sometimes severely so.

My first couple days of male menopause weren't so bad, a hot flash here and there, but nothing I couldn't live with. My initial optimism that I would be one of the lucky ones was quickly dashed as my symptoms increased markedly in strength, before culminating in the mother of all hot flashes one frigid Saturday night in the dead of a Montana January.

The barest frosting of snow lay on the dead brown grass of another dry winter. It was below zero outside but the woodstove glowed inside Greg's woodshop, where he and his brother John, fervent Dead Heads, had set up a home theater system complete with speaker tower and digital projector to show a recently remastered film of some classic old Grateful Dead concerts.

Most of the shop tools had been pushed aside, the sawdust swept away, and a dozen or so people showed up to relive a misspent youth. It was hard to watch and listen without dancing along. Before long, knees cracked and pre-arthritic arms flailed as a gaggle of fifty- and sixty-year-old baby-boomers danced on a concrete floor behind a giant table saw.

If it is unnatural for a man to go through menopause, it is doubly, no make that exponentially, unnatural for a man to go through menopause at the same time as the woman in his life. There's just too much emotional volatility. You might as well just torch a match to the gasoline and be done with it. In the past couple of days I had found myself crying for no apparent reason, and it occurred to me that this must be what two women in a relationship would endure. Dancing off by ourselves in the corner of the shop I joked to my girlfriend:

"We're like a couple of lesbians," I said.

"What!" she snapped.

"My point exactly," I replied.

Having experienced hormonal mood swings, and extrapolating to a lifetime of monthly hormonal mood swings, well, maybe I was a man who could understand. In the time it took to breathe, the thin line of belligerence that was my girlfriend's lips turned up at the corners into a slightly wicked smile.

"Can lesbians do this?" she asked.

With that she slid her hand down inside the front of my pants.

I was raised Baptist and have been trying to get over it ever since. Where I grew up holding hands was considered an untoward display of public affection; on the other hand, it was a dark room and what lesbian in his right mind would complain? If my mind was conflicted my body remained willing to rise to the occasion.

Testosterone is fundamental to this process, and chemical control centers in my hypothalamus would have been receiving a bevy of conflicting signals. Feedback loops controlling hormone levels that had worked so well for so long no longer applied. The hypothalamus is integrally tied to another part of the animal brain that processes emotions, including fear, lust, rage, and terror—any or, more likely, all of which my beast within would have been embracing at that point.

Talk about a mood swing.

"I don't feel so good," I said.

The hypothalamus is also responsible for maintaining body temperature, and the bonfire that began at the base of my skull had become a towering inferno by the time it reached my face. My girlfriend disappeared in a red mist along with everything else. I couldn't see but I could still hear, barely, as if from a great distance:

"...you feel good to me..."

I felt it coming, and I've fallen enough to know that you lead with your butt and not your head. Slump, don't topple, especially on concrete. I never completely lost consciousness although it would have been pleasant. Nobody should remember the feeling of being baked alive.

Studies have shown that, in response to the agonist I was taking, testosterone levels first climb steadily for about seven days to then spike at nearly four times baseline levels. Then, at the point receptors became desensitized, testosterone levels drop precipitously, in a matter of only a few hours, to castration levels.

I was about a week into it that night, and it is plausible that just as my body was crying out for erection fluid my hormones were instead plummeting from all time highs to all time lows. It was no wonder I was laying semi-conscious, frying in my own juices, blinded by a red mist on a concrete floor. In the distance the Grateful Dead still played; I was thinking there is no really bad time for a hand job, and wondering how I'd managed to find one, as I felt a palm on my forehead that was quickly withdrawn.

"Phew! You could cook an egg up there."

"We need to cool him down."

"What do we have?"

"Too bad there's no snow."

A group of fly-fishermen is nothing if not resourceful.

"How about we pack him in beer cans?"

The cold was exquisite. Hot flashes don't dissipate as instantaneously as they arrive but they do go. The aftermath of this flash was like the dregs of a bout with a particularly high fever. I felt seared yet purged, weak but clear. The delirium gone, I felt oddly elated. Every tumor reacts differently to hormone deprivation, and if hormone deprivation was that hard on me, it seemed certain it would be equally tough on the tumor that had sprung from me.

Die, you motherfucker, I thought, die.

Your Brain versus the Universe

From the beginning I had been determined to beat this cancer growing in my body, but would that fighting spirit help? Can the mind really influence the body in a meaningful way? And if so, how so?

In any experiment on how thoughts can affect the body there must be something to measure, and one of the factors that has been measured is hot flashes. The idea is that chemicals in the conscious mind affect chemicals in the unconscious mind, which in turn affects the concentrations of messenger chemicals in the body, which then translates into a measurable number of hot flashes.

The research also suggests it works both ways. You can think yourself into hot flashes, but you can also think yourself out of hot flashes. This is important because the chemicals behind hot flashes are the same chemicals behind stress, and the effects are far-reaching because so is the avalanche of chemical reactions your mind initiates.

In other words, no matter what you think, there you are.

Hot flashes can be used as a barometer of how minds work because your cells are designed to operate within a very specific temperature range. A fever is your body's immune response to kill bacteria that are less able to withstand a slightly higher temperature than your cells, but your body can't maintain that higher temperature for long. Outside the "normal" temperature range proteins can lose their shape and enzymes can quit working.

Too hot or too cold...your cells malfunction.

It's the same with the concentrations of potassium and glucose and all the rest of the substances of life. The levels of these chemicals in your blood must be maintained within the narrow limits of existence, and concentrations of the substances of life are controlled through the continuous interaction of the Pony Express system of messenger chemicals. It's a juggling act where the only constant is change. What goes up must come down, which is why for every chemical messenger that is an on-switch in our bodies there is also a complementary chemical off-switch.

In the case of a hot flash, two of the most potent chemicals your brain produces are involved. The hot flash off-switch is controlled by the soothing influence of opiate-like chemical messengers called *endorphins.* The on-switch is controlled by the adrenaline-based chemical norepinephrine, which your brain also produces in times of anxiety as part of the ancient fight-or-flight response.

The premise that anxiety begets norepinephrine, which begets hot flashes, was measured in a six-year study of over four hundred women published in 2005, finding that moderate and high anxiety increased hot flashes three and five times respectively over normal anxiety levels. Statistically, three-to-fivefold increases are huge, and give you some idea of the magnitude of the negative effect your brain can have on your body.

And negatively speaking, there isn't much worse than stress.

Your brain produces norepinephrine when you face physical danger, which is good, and also when you can't pay the bills or feel trapped in your job, which is bad. A checkbook isn't a man-eating tiger, it just feels like one. A fight is over quickly but money prob-lems can linger. Chronic stress leads to chronically high levels of norepinephrine, which changes what you are, and also who you are.

Too much norepinephrine for too long can make you hit the kids and kick the dog, which are not acts of which your cells are proud. It's no wonder stressed cells tend to wear out more quickly, malfunction, and perhaps even go over to the dark side of cancer. Limiting the effects of chronic stress is about as important a health step as you will ever undertake, and it can happen in two ways.

First, you can decrease production of the on-switch norepi-nephrine.

Second, you can increase production of the off-switch endor-phins.

Exercise is one of many ways you can increase your levels of en-dorphins, but this is one area where your mind can't help you. It's not enough to think about exercising, you actually have to do it, preferably until the sweat drips. Reducing levels of norepinephrine is as simple as relaxing, at least if you believe a 2005 Swedish study that examined changes in menopausal symptoms of female breast cancer survivors in response to twelve weeks of instruction in pro-gressive relaxation therapy.

Each weekly session was sixty minutes long, beginning with training in how to relax muscles in the arms, legs, face, neck, and shoulders, and progressing through whole body relaxation, cue-initiated relaxation, and differential relaxation of specific body parts. By week nine most participants had learned how to relax on demand in twenty to thirty seconds; after week twelve the women then practiced what they had learned, while recording their symptoms for a total of six months.

Over the study period, the number of hot flashes decreased from over nine per day to less than four. A standard index of overall menopausal symptoms dropped from 25.0 to 13.1. Another relaxation study showed even more striking results, with hot flash symptoms reduced by a mean of 73 percent.

Humans, using nothing more than their minds, reduced undesirable symptoms in their bodies by half to three-quarters. In terms of treatment effectiveness, those are very good numbers, much better than a lot of drugs. Plus, it's affordable, because anybody can afford to hire their own mind, and, don't forget, side effects may include a happy marriage.

If you're like me, you're thinking it's time to start paying a lot more attention to the potential healing effects of the brain, but if you're like me, you're probably not a card-carrying member of the mainstream medical establishment. The studies cited above, and many others like them, have been generally ignored as bad science.

Criticisms include factors like small sample size; there were only six women in the study that reported a 73 percent reduction in symptoms. In the applied relaxation study described above seven out of thirty-eight women dropped out for various reasons, so this study was dismissed for reasons of poor adherence to therapy. Plus, it is notoriously difficult to perform experiments on the effects of the mind in a double-blind fashion and, in today's scientific world, a study is either double-blind or it is nothing.

A study that is considered meaningful typically begins with a group of people with certain qualifications, such as women between the ages of forty and fifty with blood cholesterol over 250. The total group is then randomly assigned into subgroups, some of whom receive real treatment (such as a drug being tested to lower cholesterol), and some of whom receive sham treatment (such as a sugar pill.) Neither the people being treated nor the people giving the treatment know who is getting real treatment and who is getting sham treatment; both doctors and patients are "blind" to the truth, and hence the term *double-blind study*.

Double-blind studies are deemed necessary to account for the placebo effect, which was described in a seminal 1955 paper by an anesthesiologist named Henry Beecher. Doctor Beecher first became aware of the effect while working in military field hospitals during World War II. Morphine was in short supply and when it ran out, rather than giving a wounded soldier begging for pain relief nothing at all, Doctor Beecher injected the soldiers with saline solution and told them it was morphine.

To the doctor's astonishment, it worked.

Wounded soldiers believed the saline would relieve their pain, so it relieved their pain. Further investigation showed that, since patients could pick up on the belief of their doctor, the relative confidence of the doctor was also important in the manifestation of the placebo effect. Summing up these early findings, when doctors conveyed a belief that a medicine would work, then their patients were more likely to believe the medicine would work, which meant the medicine was far more likely to work, even if it wasn't medicine.

It was a bewildering medical development and things could have gone two ways. In one direction, the newly demonstrated power of the combined minds of the doctor-patient relationship could have been explored in depth to reveal its full potential for healing. In the other direction, the double-blind study could have been born.

And fifteen-minute office visits.

Certainly, double-blind studies to better evaluate the efficacy of new drugs are important, but the problem with applying the rigors of a double-blind study to the healing power of the mind is obvious. The placebo effect originates in the mind, and it is very difficult to design studies that are blind to the effects of a patient's own mind.

A larger question is, why would you want to?

You can't be blind to belief, and by denying data from studies that are in every way well constructed except that by their very nature they can't be double-blinded, an important part of the story as it relates to potential healing is being lost. Again sticking with hot flashes as an example of how this can happen, consider a sweeping 2006 paper that reviewed the available literature on complementary and alternative therapies for the management of menopause-related symptoms.

Five data bases, collectively citing over 13.5 million abstracts and articles, were searched, yielding a total of 1,432 abstracts that met study criteria. After review of the abstracts, 1,249 of the studies were rejected, leaving 183 studies in which the full articles were read. After review, 113 of these articles were rejected, leaving a total of 70 articles for inclusion in the study paper. Of the 70 studies that made the final cut, 35 were regarded to be of poor quality with suspect results, leaving 35 studies that were ultimately deemed inconclusive, leading to the conclusion that complementary and alternative therapies showed little benefit in treating menopausal symptoms.

This could be interpreted as a rigorous review that protects the interests of the patients, or it could be the baby just got tossed out with the bath water. Either way, the double-blind mandate drastically affects what health information trickles down to the public, as does the vast amount of money involved.

To see how this might work, consider a 2002 review on the cause and potential treatment of hot flashes that cited 112 papers covering a variety of alternative treatments, including the effects of soy, a flower (black cohosh) in the buttercup family, red clover, vitamin E, relaxation training, paced respiration, exercise, and counseling. All these treatments have shown significant reductions in hot flashes in some studies, but not all, which led researchers to recommend—surprise—prescription drugs for severe symptoms.

These drugs are a developing class of antidepressants that affect the reuptake of endorphins and norepinephrine in the hypothalamus. The drugs did reduce hot flash symptoms, about as effectively as the earlier reported relaxation techniques. The drugs also display a rich array of all the side effects you would expect of antidepressants, and one side effect you may not have anticipated, which is that a new use for a drug that is already FDA approved is a pharmaceutical company's wet dream.

Half the people on the planet go through menopause.

Billions are at stake.

As I review the literature, with no vested interest other than trying to live a couple more years, it's like it's been decided by somebody somewhere that it's cheating to use your mind to heal. You're supposed to get better in spite of the placebo effect, not in addition to it. Virtually every clinical trial over the last fifty years documents that placebos help a significant number of people who take them, yet doctors are understandably reluctant to prescribe placebos.

Ethically, a doctor in good faith can't give someone a sugar pill. Even if it worked, a thousand lawyers would be lined up waiting to sue for malpractice, which brings up the question as to why the sugar pill is necessary in the first place.

It isn't the sugar pill that does the work, it's our minds. The chicanery of a placebo isn't necessary for our minds to affect our bodies, yet the great bulk of the research in this direction assumes that without the placebo there can be no placebo effect. This attitude is slowly changing, and slow is OK, unless you're running out of time.

I could live with hot flashes.

The question was whether I would live at all.

It's one thing to believe my mind could control the production of the chemicals that caused hot flashes, and because I believed it would work it was more likely to work, but it's another thing entirely that my mind might help kill off an existing tumor. Or is it? Conventional medical wisdom ridicules the idea that we can think our way out of a tumor, but could there be some brain-body link that would at least enable my mind to join in the fight against the cancer I already had?

In fact, there is a great deal of evidence that the same chemicals behind hot flashes and stress also exert powerful influences on your body's immune response, including the production of natural killer cells, your best internal defense against existing cancer cells. If we can think our way out of hot flashes there is every reason to believe we can likewise stimulate our immune systems. This is something I learned a little later in the game, and is covered in more detail in a later chapter but, for now, consider this:

It's unlikely you'll be a success in this life unless you believe you'll be a success in this life. You won't be a winner unless you believe you can be a winner. All those gold medalists standing on the dais at the Olympics, none of them say, "I got here because I didn't think I could do it. I just never thought I could be a champion, and therefore I never tried. I didn't practice, I didn't sacrifice, I just didn't care."

It seems, to me, it's the same with cancer.

If you don't believe you can beat it, you're probably right.

Doctor Dilemma

I, along with most of my generation, grew up thinking doctors were infallible. Doctors weren't like fishing guides and plumbers and tax accountants. I didn't figure doctors made mistakes like the rest of us, but, in this, I was simply naive, and I wondered how I could have missed so much for so long as my investigation into health care led me to the topic of iatrogenic death.

Iatrogenic is a word that refers to the inadvertent effects of medical treatment; death is self explanatory. Simply put, this category includes all the people who enter willingly into treatments they expect will make them better, but instead the treatments make them dead. It wasn't much discussed until the shit hit the bedpan in 1999 with the publication of an Institute of Health paper called "To Err is Human," which estimated that 44,000 to 98,000 Americans died each year as a direct result of medical error.

"Oops...sorry...but you're dead."

A commentary on this 1999 report published the next year in the *Journal of the American Medical Association* estimated total iatrogenic deaths, not just the ones due to demonstrable error, at somewhere from 225,000 to 284,000. Do the math, this leaves somewhere between 127,000 and 240,000 additional Americans dying annually of medical treatments that were deemed to have been correctly prescribed.

"Oops...sorry...it worked on the last guy."

Of course, you may wonder why a treatment isn't a mistake if it kills you, but there you have it. Even at the low end of 225,000 iatrogenic deaths per year, this estimate makes medical care the third leading cause of mortality in the United States, and nearly all assessments of iatrogenic issues agree it is a hugely underreported problem.

So, as bad as this sounds, it's probably worse.

A high proportion of the listed causes of iatrogenic death include the wrong drug being prescribed, and side effects from the right drug being prescribed. In either case the Pony Express system of messenger chemicals is affected to the point that your body can no longer keep you alive. The problem is compounded by chemical cocktails; the pushing and pulling of various drugs simply overwhelms your system.

Unnecessary surgeries, unnecessary hospitalizations, unnecessary diagnostic procedures, and antibiotic-resistant infections are all part of the iatrogenic whole. As an example, a woman I know broke her leg. Complications ensued, including a staph infection, for which she was hospitalized and placed on potent antibiotics.

The antibiotics interfered with the normal working of the digestive bacteria in her intestines, and she now has a serious disease of the colon to go with her staph infection. Plus, during her lengthy hospitalization, as a cost-cutting measure, the hospital changed the policy on doctors.

No longer does a patient see a single doctor. Instead, a rotating team of doctors comes through. Whatever benefit there might be in a strong doctor-patient relationship has been lost and, with each new doctor, each with a new opinion, the chance of mistakes and undesirable pharmaceutical interactions increases.

That'll teach you to break your leg.

About the only area in which the United States ranks first in world health care is in the amount we spend, at over 15 percent of the gross domestic product, or over two trillion dollars. This far exceeds what any other country spends on health care, and it doesn't buy much. A report by the World Health Organization in the year 2000 ranked America 72nd out of 191 countries in the overall performance of health care; another study on health care ranked the United States 15th out of 25 industrialized countries.

To put it bluntly, "Huh?"

How could this be? And where did all that money go?

Well, part of it goes to politicians who deny this money affects their votes to pass laws favorable to the medical industry, and part of it goes to publicity that had always kept me convinced American health care was the best in the world. Many powerful medical entities have a vested interest in disputing iatrogenic issues, but that doesn't make the dangers any less real, and this topic more than anything else made me realize how important it was that I take charge of my own health care.

There is an educational bias among conventional physicians toward the use of powerful pharmaceuticals and invasive diagnostic procedures, and this bias is reinforced by the threat of malpractice suits. When you walk through those hospital doors, custom, ethics, and past lawsuits dictate that in the name of treatment your cells are about to encounter a wide variety of situations they have never encountered before, some of which are as likely to kill them as help them.

That's just the way it is.

Medical diagnosis and subsequent treatment is both art and science tempered with experience. There's some educated guesswork involved, some hunches to play, and nobody knows your body better than you. It's OK to disagree with your doctor, to err on the side of fewer pills and procedures rather than more, to take it slowly, but if you do, side effects can include the fact that you have to get a new doctor.

I went through a few doctors. There were plenty of good ones, but it was tough finding anybody with whom I was on the same wavelength, and this applied to matters as basic as diet. It depends on the school, but I've read that medical students typically spend only a week or two on diet, if that. Again, there's that educational bias.

Plus, the evidence on the cancer-fighting power of food is so contradictory that it's safer to recommend nothing rather than something. Out of the ten doctors I talked to only one had much of anything to say about the benefits of diet, but even that was more of an aside. His main area of expertise was radiation, a topic in which my cells were very much interested, because, let's face it: atomic bombs can be detrimental to your health.

My conventional treatments would include the implantation of tiny radioactive pellets called *seeds* directly into my main tumor. I wanted whoever did that to be among the very best at what they did, and I felt very fortunate indeed to be able to drive the five hundred miles it took to fit into the busy schedule of a highly-skilled practitioner in the art of radioactive implants we'll call Doctor Seed.

I'd had a couple of sour doctor experiences. One became incensed when I asked for my records to get a second opinion; another blew me off in fifteen minutes after I'd traveled two days to see him. It was more of an insult than an appointment. But with Doctor Seed, our patient/physician karma was good from the start.

For one thing, Doctor Seed had read one of my fly-fishing books. I felt like more than just a name on a chart, and on top of that, he cared. His credentials as an expert in his field were formidable, and my confidence in his knowledge was cemented ten minutes into our consultation when a nurse stuck her head in the door.

"It's Doctor So-and-so," she said, "from Berlin."

"Berlin?" I said. "Germany?"

Doctor Seed nodded apologetically.

"I'll be right back," he said. "But I really should take this call."

He'd return, we'd talk, and then the nurse would stick her head in the door.

"It's Doctor So-and-so," she'd say, "from Chicago."

It went that way the entire time I was in his office; clearly Doctor Seed had bigger fish to fry than a trout guide from Montana. My hour and a half of questions took nearly three hours to answer, but I never felt that he begrudged the time it took to answer questions he must have answered time and time again.

"I understand we have to kill the tumor," I said. "But still, I'm worried about the effects of radiation on my healthy cells…"

"Healthy cells will die but cancer cells divide more rapidly than normal cells and are less adept at repairing the damage that radiation causes; therefore radiation is more likely to kill cancerous cells than damage healthy cells."

My rectal cells were among those especially pleased by that news.

"Do you do the surgery yourself?"

"Absolutely."

"How many of these seed implant surgeries have you done? "Thousands."

Now there was a guy I could believe in, and believe I did as we went over the details of my conventional treatment. At the time of this appointment it had been about ten weeks since my diagnosis with cancer, and for the first time I allowed myself some hope as I asked the biggest question of all.

"So, what are my chances…realistically?"

I wiped the sweat of a juicy hot flash from my brow and stared at Doctor Seed, who scratched at his beard as he turned to stare out the window at the tall buildings. A guy like that, he wouldn't even lie about the size of the trout he caught, which is probably why he avoided my question as he turned back from the window.

"You should continue to live your life as if you'll continue to live your life," he said, "but at the same time it would be well to put your affairs in order."

Sometimes it's tough to swallow good advice.

Doctor Seed was an expert in the field of radiation, and also a Doctor of Osteopathy. Generally, an osteopath undergoes the same medical school and residency training as an M.D., but also takes an additional three hundred to five hundred hours in the study of hands-on manual medicine and the body's musculoskeletal system. Osteopaths tend to see healing as a process that involves the body as a whole, and in a book he'd written Doctor Seed had a whole chapter summarizing recent research into how diet might be a factor in the prevention and treatment of cancer.

Again, here was a guy I could believe in.

"So what should I eat?" I asked.

"Flaxseed oil and soy products," he said.

"And what should I avoid?"

"Saturated fats," he said.

It wasn't the first time I'd heard saturated fats were bad for me, but it was the first time I bothered to find out if it was true.

The Skinny on Fats

If iatrogenic issues were the most sobering topic I researched, then fats were the most illuminating. I did not understand how diet could affect cancer until I understood fats, and if you want to understand fats, it's back to a bit of chemistry.

Don't panic, it's organic.

Organic molecules, including fats, contain carbon, the fourth most abundant element in the universe and, at about 18.5 percent by weight, the second most abundant element in the human body. Carbon, the sixth element in the periodic table, is comprised of a nucleus of six protons and (usually) six neutrons surrounded by a total of six whirring electrons. Two of these electrons fill the inner energy shell, while the outer, or valence, electron shell of carbon is exactly half full with four electrons.

The forces that drive the universe are satisfied only when the second shell of an atom is full with eight electrons. This makes carbon, with four valence electrons, a convivial atom that can form bonds with up to four other atoms at a time, and part and parcel to over ten million known compounds. From gases to metals, carbon willingly enters into covalent relationships with a host of other elements, including itself, all of which makes carbon the life of the molecular party.

Literally.

Rings and strings of carbon atoms provide the frameworks that make the organic chemistry of life possible. When these carbon atoms share electrons with hydrogen atoms, the resulting molecules are called, obviously enough, hydrocarbons. If you looked at it in terms of the electron dance at the Atomic Ball, then carbon is among the luckiest of atoms, because it can dance with up to four partners at once, and if I can't be a carbon, I'm content that I at least have some in me.

One dance that has been popular among hydrocarbons on the planet Earth since the days of primordial soup is an old-fashioned line dance in which a string of carbon atoms is sandwiched between, and shares electrons with, two strings of hydrogen atoms. The result of all this covalent mingling is full valence shells all around, except for the carbon atoms at each end of the line, which each still need one electron. When this electron is provided by another hydrogen atom at one end, and by an oxygen-rich carboxyl group at the other end, then you have the molecule called a fatty acid.

Fatty acids are essential to cellular life and are pictured on the following page; the three-hydrogen end turns out to be a very stable arrangement. It's almost impossible to break up, like a fifties sitcom family. Imagine June Cleaver having an affair. It's just not going to happen. The carboxyl group, on the other hand, is more like a Desperate Housewife. A carboxyl group is the active end of a fatty acid, with promiscuous oxygen atoms that can't help but jump into relationships with other electrons.

When the carbon atoms in the middle of a fatty acid string each share one electron, then each carbon gets two electrons, one from each side. Each carbon still needs two electrons, and in one particularly stable arrangement those missing electrons can be supplied by two hydrogen atoms. The carbon chain is said to be

Common Fatty Acids

| Saturated Palmitic Acid | Omega-9 Oleic Acid | Omega-6 Linoleic Acid | Omega-3 Linolenic Acid |

C is Carbon, H is Hydrogen, O is Oxygen, and the lines between atoms denote the sharing of electrons through either single or double covalent bonds. The branched carbon-oxygen-oxygen-hydrogen group at the top of each hydrocarbon chain denotes a carboxyl group, the active group that allows fatty acids to react with molecules of glycerine to form triglycerides. The number of double carbon bonds, with the associated missing hydrogen atoms, a seemingly minor difference, is what gives these fatty acids their distinctive biologic properties, and each of these fatty acids plays crucial roles in your overall health. You don't need just one or the other, you need them all.

saturated in hydrogen, because there isn't any room for more electrical partners, and this is what we call a saturated fatty acid.

A saturated fatty acid is a symmetrical molecule with balanced
forces. It lays out in a line like a ladder, and linear molecules can
pack together more closely at any given temperature than curved
molecules. This is why saturated fats are solid at room temperature, and it's a good thing. Otherwise our breasts and buttocks
would drip out of our bras and pants, and who needs that, unless
you own a paper towel plant.

If the specifics of all this covalent bonding stuff are confusing
don't worry about it. Our electrons know what they're doing and,
just as carbon atoms in a string can share one electron, at certain
places in the string they can also share two electrons.

This sharing of one extra electron between carbon atoms eliminates the need for two hydrogen atoms (go figure), and the fatty
acid is now said to be unsaturated in hydrogen. It's a different kind
of love, and since there are less overall electrons to go around, carbon atoms involved in double covalent bonds are more likely to
look outside the relationship for new partners with more electrons. It's the same old story.

If your needs aren't being completely satisfied at home…

That's chemistry.

Unsaturated fats can be monounsaturated, meaning they have
one double carbon bond and two missing hydrogen atoms, or
polyunsaturated, meaning they have more than one double carbon
bond and an equivalent number of missing pairs of hydrogen
atoms. Each of these unshielded-by-hydrogen double carbon
bonds is more prone to interaction with outside electrical partners, and oxygen is one atom in particular that does not like to
take no for an answer. Light and heat both encourage the transfer
of electrons through the process of oxidation at these double carbon bonds; it is oxidation that causes oils to go rancid, and this is

why unsaturated oils are best stored in sealed, dark bottles in cool, dark places.

Familiar fatty acids can range from four to twenty-four carbon atoms long. A string of four carbon atoms saturated in hydrogen is what flavors butter, a string of twenty-two carbon atoms with six double bonds is common in coldwater fish, and the reactive characteristics of each fatty acid vary greatly depending on the nature of the carbon strings on which they are based.

Three unsaturated fatty acids built on a chain of eighteen carbon atoms get a lot of press. The location and number of the double bonds make every unsaturated fatty acid chemically unique, and scientists describe the location of these double bonds by counting up from the last carbon at the unreactive end of the string. Medical scientists also have an affinity for the Greek language that probably dates back to Hippocrates, and since the last letter in the Greek alphabet is omega, then the last carbon at the end of the string is also called the *omega*.

Count up nine carbons from the end of an eighteen-carbon string and stick in a double bond; you have omega-9 oleic acid, the main oil in both olives and your skin. Add another double bond between the sixth and seventh carbon atoms, for a total of two double bonds and four missing hydrogen atoms, and you have linoleic acid, an omega-6 oil found concentrated in the seeds of grapes. Add another double bond at carbon atom number three, for a total of three double bonds and six missing hydrogen atoms, and you have linolenic acid, the omega-3 fatty acid found concentrated in flax seeds.

The omega-6 linoleic and the omega-3 linolenic fatty acids are also called *essential fatty acids* because, like vitamins, although these compounds are essential to your life, your body can't manufacture them. Essential fatty acids you have to eat, and no fatty acid tends to exist individually on Earth.

The carboxyl group at the active end of the carbon chain dangles electrons like bait. There are plenty of molecules eager to snap up this bait, including glycerol, which, by virtue of its particular arrangement of semilinear atoms, can share electrons with not one but three fatty acids. The result of all these mingled electrons is three fatty acids hanging like wagging tails from a molecular stick of glycerol; the combination is described as a triglyceride.

Triglycerides, and their constituent fatty acids, form a dominant functional component of plant and animal cells. They're critically important, and you might think, as I thought, that a triglyceride would be all one fat or the other. The dangling fatty acids would either be all saturated, or they would be all unsaturated, because otherwise how could you avoid "bad" saturated fats while maximizing "good" unsaturated fats?

The simple truth is you can't.

You're not supposed to, not if you want to stay healthy. This is nature's lesson. We need all these fatty acids, not just some of them. Natural triglycerides mix fatty acids, pretty much all the time, every time. Take a typical bottle of olive oil for instance.

The exact composition of that oil depends on genetics, soils, weather, and time of harvest, but a mean fatty acid analysis of 78 Greek virgin olive oils (the oils produced from the first press of raw olives) showed *thirteen* different fatty acids were present, dominated by omega-9 oleic acid (77 percent), saturated palmitic acid (10.5 percent), omega-6 linoleic acid (7.5 percent), and 5 percent everything else, including several antioxidants. Unprocessed palm oil, since 2004 the most widely distributed commodity oil worldwide, typically has concentrations of 45 percent saturated palmitic acid, 40 percent omega-9 oleic acid, 10 percent omega-6 linoleic acid, and 5 percent all kinds of other nutrients, including carotene. Even pork lard is generally only 42 percent saturated fat (in a combination of several saturated fatty acids), 44 percent omega-9 oleic acid, 10 percent omega-6 linoleic acid, and 4 percent other important nutrients.

As humans, we need all kinds of fatty acids, for all kinds of reasons.

Forget that tripe that saturated fats are bad for you. After more than fifty years of research, after tens of thousands of studies, the conclusive evidence just isn't there. Let common sense prevail. We, as humans, are saturated fat. We're other things too, but without fat we would collapse into puddles of protein-soluble water. Each of the various fatty acids are incorporated into molecules with specific functions in our bodies, some major, some minor, but all essential to the process we call life.

The television tells you otherwise, but it's ridiculous to pretend we can improve our health by eating a lot of one fatty acid and none of another. Our cells simply don't work that way. We need fats, a lot of different fats, but, that said, too much fat is just as bad for you as too little. It isn't a question of unsaturated or saturated, it's a question of excessive caloric intake.

A gram of any fat contains nine calories of energy, a gram of carbohydrate or protein four calories. For a medieval peasant trying to survive the Little Ice Age in a grass thatched hovel of sticks, the extra energy in the fat of the milk from his cow's teat could very well have been the difference between life and death. For a contemporary desk jockey who counts walking to the vending machine as exercise, the cumulative store of extra energy in the fat of a milk chocolate habit can also be the difference between life and death, this time from obesity.

No study says being obese is good for you. On this point the science is clear: too much fat will kill you just as dead as too little fat, with side effects including either a big urn or a jumbo coffin.

Fear of Frying

The benign relationship between humans and their fats took a detour in the year 1902, when a patent for the hydrogenation of liquid oils was granted to the German scientist Wilheim Normann. Herr Normann discovered that cooking unsaturated fatty acids at high temperatures in the presence of pressurized hydrogen and a catalyst such as platinum could break apart the double carbon bonds, force hydrogen atoms into the crack in the molecule, and create a single carbon bond saturated in hydrogen atoms.

Unsaturated fats cooked until every unsaturated double bond is replaced with a saturated single bond are completely hydrogenated oils. The problem is exactly that: these fats are completely saturated. Even butter is only 50 percent saturated fat, including several different saturated fatty acids of varying numbers of carbon atoms in length. In oil cooked to complete hydrogenation, on the other hand, all the fatty acid carbon chains are saturated in hydrogen, and most of the chains are eighteen carbon atoms long.

It's too much of one thing. You lose the health-giving variety of fatty acids in the triglycerides typically found in nature, but at least your body can digest completely hydrogenated oils. Partially hydrogenated oils are a different story.

During partial hydrogenation some of the double carbon bonds that are broken then reform not as a single carbon bond saturated in hydrogen, but as another double carbon bond. These double carbon bonds are directional, and can reform in one of two ways: with the hydrogen atoms on the same side of the carbon chain, or with hydrogen atoms on opposite sides of the carbon chain.

The double bonds in unsaturated fats found in nature, with a few exceptions found mostly in ruminants such as cows, have the hydrogen atoms lined up on the same side of the carbon chain in a *cis* bond (from Latin for *same*). This atomic structure causes the carbon chain to bend at the double bond. The more double bonds there are, the more the fatty acid bends, and, from simple curves to molecules that look like double-jointed fish hooks, your cells use all of these different shapes in specific ways.

The Latin word for *across* or *opposite* is *trans*. A *trans fat* is one in which the hydrogen atoms in an unsaturated double carbon bond are found across from each other. A trans bond does not bend like a cis bond. A trans fatty acid is straight but, since it's missing hydrogen atoms, your cells interpret it as curved.

It would be like you're building a house and every time you called for a window you got a piece of plywood instead, but you didn't know you'd been tricked. As far as you could tell you were getting windows, and it's dark inside the house. You need light to restore the balance. You keep calling for more windows, but the more fake windows you put up, the darker it gets, and before long the house becomes unusable.

That is the effect of trans fats on your cells. Your cells are constantly calling for parts to adjust the dynamic equilibrium of cellular balances. When they call for curves and are fooled by lines the dynamic equilibrium of life quickly goes awry, and your cells don't know why. Building techniques that worked just fine for billions

TRANS FATS

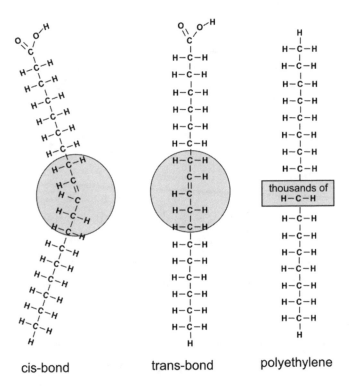

cis-bond   trans-bond   polyethylene

The difference is the location of a single hydrogen atom, but a a cis bond bends while a trans bond doesn't. It may not seem like much, but it's the difference between a line and a curve, and curves do things lines can't. For instance, nobody ever got back to where they started by going in a straight line, and nobody ever got ahead by going in a circle. The difference is as fundamental as the geometrical grid upon which our universe is built.

Your body recognizes trans fat as unsaturated fat because of its missing hydrogen atoms, yet due to its straight shape trans fat will not enter into normal reactions with enzymes in your body. Trans fat behaves more like the polymer polyethylene, the common and nonbiodegradable plastic that is found in everything from milk jugs to kevlar.

of years no longer apply, and this is now a cell that is primed for trouble.

As one example of troubled cells, consider that fatty acids pushed up one against the next are a primary component of your semipermeable cell membranes. This permeability must be controlled within the limits of life, and curved fatty acids can't pack as tightly together as straight fatty acids. It's like trying to pack a room full of people, some with their arms sticking out and some with their arms at their sides.

It's a tough go squeezing through a crowd packed tightly together with their arms at their sides. It's the cellular equivalent of reducing permeability, and oxygen likewise has a tough go of squeezing through tightly packed fatty acids. When oxygen levels drop your cells call for more curved fatty acids to increase permeability, but if they get straight trans bonds instead of curved cis bonds, then permeability decreases rather than increases. There's less oxygen instead of more, creating cellular energy deficits that can lead to cellular dedifferentiation and cancer.

As originally conceived, hydrogenated oils were meant to be used in the manufacture of soap, but the market never developed. If money was to be made another avenue was required, and since these altered oils packed together tightly enough to be solid at room temperature, some marketing genius had the bright idea to use them to replace the butter and lard in baked goods.

From soap to cupcakes, that's m-m-m good.

Crisco, the first shortening to be made entirely of hydrogenated vegetable oils, was introduced in 1911 and touted as an economic alternative that would revolutionize the American kitchen. It truly was a remarkable new substance, as shown by the original 1912 advertising, which had this to say: "You can fry fish in Crisco, and the Crisco will not absorb the fish odor! You can then use the same

Crisco for frying potatoes without imparting to them the slightest fish flavor."

The fact that even fish oil didn't enter into molecular relationships with trans fats should have been a tip-off. However, this was the cutting edge of modern living and, then as now, consumers jumped on the bandwagon. Cookbooks were produced and distributed free of charge, every recipe calling for liberal doses of this miraculous white gel that made such fine pie crusts and airy dumplings. Home economists were hired to teach the use of Crisco in cooking schools around the country, and thus began a parade of ballyhooed products containing trans fats that could be kept palatable for years.

The use of partially hydrogenated oils increased steadily until World War II, when sales rose sharply as Americans adapted to butter rationing by switching over to margarine. In 1957 the American Heart Association first proposed that a diet high in saturated fats could lead to increased risk of heart disease, thus ushering in the golden age of trans fats. Over most of the next four decades partially hydrogenated oils became nearly ubiquitous in processed and restaurant foods as saturated fats were increasingly vilified. Yet, despite this noble effort by the food industry to minimize natural fats in the diet, heart disease remained at epidemic proportions in America.

What could be wrong?

Thousands of studies had been funded and conducted. Billions had been spent to study the effects of fat on human health, yet after nearly fifty years of research there was virtually no data that separated the effects of trans fats from naturally occurring fats. The real world is a complex continuum of cause and effect. It is a major flaw in the nature of contemporary reductionist research that scientists, in focusing intently on the effects of whatever variable they have chosen to examine in their particular study, often miss the effects of other variables and how those variables interact to form a whole.

It wasn't until the 1990s, to the dismay of a food industry grown increasingly reliant on partially hydrogenated oils, that facts on the deleterious effects of trans fats on human health began to gain serious attention. An avalanche of corroborating studies on the dangers of artificially hydrogenated oils finally led the United States Food and Drug Administration (FDA) to require that food manufacturers, beginning in 2006, list the amount of trans fat in the products they sell.

This should have made it at least possible to avoid dietary trans fats, but the FDA, in collaboration with the food industry, left loopholes big enough to drive a hearse through. One caveat in the legislation is that foods containing less than 0.5 grams per serving can be listed as containing 0 (zero) grams on the nutrition facts panel.

So, by changing the serving size, trans-fat-rich foods can be passed off as trans-fat-free foods. This is why the same label may say in big letters at the top that a product contains zero grams of trans fat per serving, while at the same time listing hydrogenated oil, partially hydrogenated oil, or shortening (the legal euphemisms for trans fat) in the fine print of the list of ingredients at the bottom of the label.

No wonder it's confusing.

I'm from the government and I'm here to help you.

As a further example of how the FDA has our backs, consider that the difference between monoglycerides, diglycerides, and triglycerides is simply whether one, two, or three fatty acid tails hang from a molecule of glycerine. However, since mono- and diglycerides are defined as emulsifiers rather than fats, only the trans fatty acids in triglycerides have to be reported. The point of all this is that vast quantities of trans fats are hiding all over our grocery shelves and, if you care about what you eat, when it comes to processed foods, you can't tell what you're eating.

Abundant evidence says eating as little as two grams of trans fat a day imparts very significant health risks, yet the average daily intake of trans fat for Americans twenty years of age and older in 2008 was estimated at 5.8 grams, with the 90th percentile at 9.4 grams. In another study, an analysis of U.S. food between 2005 and 2008 found 20 grams of trans fat in a typical fast food meal, while a four ounce serving of microwave popcorn or crackers contained 12 and 15 grams of trans fat respectively.

Think you aren't typical?

Well, neither did I.

I thought I ate pretty healthily, but I was gobbling trans fats from day one. There were partially hydrogenated oils in my infant formula, in the jars of baby food, and in the cereals, bread, margarine, and peanut butter that my teeth later allowed me to eat. We ate what the black-and-white TV told us to eat, and in my family, especially for Mom because it was a night she didn't have to cook, McFood was a McTreat.

It's a tradition I carried on with my kids, in part because they clamored to go to a restaurant that featured giant slides and pits full of play balls. In we'd go, and when we left, we'd be carrying a couple ounces of trans fats between us. As part of my anticancer regimen I quit (mostly) eating processed foods. I looked at it like chemotherapy, only tasty, but in all those prior decades, at 5 to 10 grams a day, I figure I ate somewhere between two and four hundred pounds of trans fats…at least.

So where did it all go?

It went somewhere because I don't weigh four hundred pounds, but it didn't go easily. The evidence is meager and conflicting on how our bodies metabolize trans fats, but it is clear that trans fats persist in our cells for the same reason foods built from trans fats persist without spoiling. Carrots rot, Twinkies don't. With trans fats, what was once a relatively weak cis covalent bond, susceptible to reaction with other molecules in the process of life, now resembles in form and function some of the longest-lived molecules on Earth, polyethylene plastics.

Polyethylene, the polymer behind everything from milk jugs to artificial hips, like natural fatty acids, is a linear hydrocarbon chain. Polyethylene differs from nature's fats in that the carbon chain is much longer and both ends are capped with unreactive hydrogen atoms. What this carbon chain has in common with trans fats is that the digestive enzymes of life don't tend to recognize either of these particular molecular sequences as food.

They're non-biodegradable substances. Trans fats don't spoil for much the same reasons polyethylene takes centuries for nature to break down. At the level of covalent bonds, chemical reactions don't occur. The electrons don't dance, and, to visualize the cumulative effects of trans fats in our bodies, consider that any realistic seascape of any shore on any ocean now includes an array of vividly colored plastics that date back to the buckets I used for building sand castles on the shores of Lake Erie.

High density polyethylene, the backbone of most plastic containers, was first produced on a large-scale commercial basis beginning in 1954, the same year I was born. Fifty-five years later just one island of floating plastic in the eastern Pacific Ocean is estimated to be as much as twice the size of the continental United States, and the American Cancer Society now reports one out of two men and one out of three women will come down with cancer.

Increasing evidence appears to show there isn't an upper end to the detrimental effects of trans fats. The more you eat, the worse it is. On the other hand, trans fatty acids do have an active end, and even though enzymes don't tend to recognize these artificial fats, the carbon chains do eventually oxidize, perhaps in much the same way you can get rid of polyethylene by burning it, if you don't mind the smell.

The true nature of trans fats was brought home to me one day deep in the heart of Ascension Bay in southern Mexico. I was working at the Pesca Maya Fishing Lodge, teaching a class on how to be better fly-fishing guides to a group of Mayan Indians, and we pulled up in our boat at an island in the middle of the bay for lunch. This particular island has a resident colony of iguanas, and these lizards are used to being fed.

Felipe, the patriarch of a local Mayan clan, had lived in the area his entire life. He threw bread, processed lunch meat, tomatoes, lettuce, and apples up on the spit of sand at the edge of the shore; the lizards ate it all. Finally, it was time for dessert.

"Will they eat the cookies?" I asked.

You haven't had junk food until you've had third world junk food; the cookies were florescent pink and white marshmallow gobs so rich in high fructose corn syrup it made your teeth hurt just looking at them.

"*Su favorito*," said Felipe. "Their favorite."

Sugar is indeed the universal foodstuff, and the boss iguana, a good two feet long, snapped up a tossed cookie and scuttled off with his treasure, his lips glued together with pink marshmallow jutting out from either side of his narrow jaw.

"And what about this?" I asked.

The last item on the menu came in foil pouches and looked like fried pretzels.

Felipe shrugged his big round shoulders.

"*No lo comen*," he said. "They won't eat it."

Finding it hard to believe that lizards on a mangrove island in the middle of the ocean wouldn't eat any human food that came their way, I tossed some pretzels up on the sand. No matter how many pretzels I threw, the iguanas paid the decorative brown curls no more mind than they paid the plastic bottles that had washed up on shore.

What's in this stuff? I wondered.

The list of ingredients on the pretzel label was quite short and included, in order of abundance, partially hydrogenated oils, refined flour, and preservatives. This truly was an entrée for the apocalypse, and it seems reasonable to assume that if stranded lizards don't recognize trans fats as food, you shouldn't either.

Bound by the Chains
of Scientific Dogma

My observations of the lizards constitute what scientists call anecdotal evidence. It's an unsubstantiated story. The sample size was small, including only a dozen or so iguanas, and peer review was limited to a couple of seagulls and a vulture. The results from this simple experiment are potentially misleading, which points out the greater and largely ignored truth that the results from all experiments are potentially misleading, and this is particularly true of data drawn from epidemiological studies.

Epidemiology is the study of the incidence and distribution of disease in various populations, with an eye toward relating differences in disease rates to some root cause. The idea that diet affects health goes back at least as far as Hippocrates and the ancient Greeks, but Doctor Ancel Keys is generally regarded as a pioneer in the design of large scale epidemiological studies that explore the associations between diet and disease in contrasting populations of people.

Doctor Keys, during World War II, noticed that levels of heart attacks dropped significantly in food deprived European populations. His own work in Minnesota found an "epidemic" of heart attacks in well-to-do executives; European physicians revealed they too saw high levels of heart attacks in affluent clientele. A peripatetic scientist, Doctor Keys became convinced during his travels in the 1950s that first, different countries had statistically significant differences in heart disease, second, these differences were likely due to diet, and third, cholesterol was somehow involved.

The third assumption had roots in a widely reported story about a Wisconsin dairy farmer who was referred to Key's laboratory. This farmer had large knobs on his elbows and above his eyes, knobs that when surgically opened proved to be composed nearly entirely of pure yellow waxy cholesterol. The farmer's blood serum cholesterol reading was over one thousand, so, as a simple experiment, just to see what would happen, the scientists put the farmer on a fat free diet.

"Bang!" goes the anecdote, after one week of a fat free diet the farmer's blood cholesterol level had halved to five hundred. When the farmer was fed fat in the form of margarine, which is actually trans fat, cholesterol levels shot back up. This research was performed in a facility so underfunded it was located beneath the bleachers of the football stadium, and was among the experiments that led to the hypothesis that diets high in fat cause blood serum high in cholesterol, which in turn causes heart disease.

Doctor Keys set out to objectively prove these subjective impressions with the Seven Countries Study, an ambitious project far beyond the scope of anything that had ever been tried before. Enlisting the aid of a community of internationally respected scientists, with an initial budget from a central grant that averaged only $25,000 per year per study area, systematic surveys were taken between 1958 and 1970 of men aged 40-59 in eighteen areas of seven countries: Yugoslavia, Italy, Greece, Finland, the Netherlands, the United States, and Japan.

Epidemiological study groups need to show consistent dietary trends within a given population, and dietary diversity between populations. It was decided groups of working-class men in rural areas best met these criteria, and dietary contrasts between groups indeed proved significant. From one country to the next, levels of daily saturated fat consumption varied from 3 to 22 percent, total dietary fat intake ranged from 9 to 40 percent of daily calories, and cholesterol levels in the blood of Finnish loggers and Japanese fishermen showed almost no overlap.

Study populations also showed high variation in rates of coronary disease. The extremes came in the Greek island of Crete and eastern Finland. For every rural Cretan man dying of heart disease there were over one hundred eastern Finnish loggers, and more than simple nuance distinguished typical meals between these two countries.

Doctor Henry Blackburn, the first project director for the Seven Countries Study, described the Finnish loggers' lunches as "things of wonder, unsurpassed in caloric density. Large hunks of meat are suspended in congealed fat, enveloped in a dark bread loaf fully permeated by fat. The whole—at 250 grams of fat and well over 2,000 calories—is packaged in aluminum foil and tied with a ribbon."

And that's just lunch. For snacks it was customary to butter cheese, and we're talking my ancestors here. I'm one-quarter Finnish on my father's mother's side. Cheese isn't just a birthright, it's my heritage.

The Finnish loggers in the Seven Countries Study, despite their predilection for saturated fat, were to all outward appearances strong, lean, and fit. Yet, as far as heart attacks went, they were tree-cutting time bombs. This was in stark contrast to the Greek island of Crete, where rural men generally worked in the vineyards or olive groves.

At the time, in the early sixties, Cretan men walked or rode bicycles to work. Televisions were rare, electricity new. Grain was winnowed in stone circles, as opposed to bleached in vats. Typical meals were high in fruits, vegetables, grains, legumes, complex carbohydrates, and fibers. Red wine, one of my favorite food groups, made regular mealtime appearances, while meats such as lamb (naturally spiced from grazing in thyme filled fields) might be eaten once a week, chicken once a week, and fresh caught fish a couple times a week.

Overall fat consumption remained high in Crete, mostly due to high levels of dietary olive oil, yet heart disease and blood cholesterol remained low. Overall fat consumption was similarly high in Finland, mostly due to meat and dairy products, yet blood cholesterol and heart disease was high. The researchers applied the methods of covariant analysis to this conundrum, and concluded, reasonably, that saturated fatty acids characteristic of meat and dairy products were associated with high cholesterol and heart disease, while the monounsaturated fatty acids typical of olive oil weren't.

For the first time a link between heart disease, cholesterol, and saturated fats had been "proven." Entire industries sprang up, and once a pharmaceutical industry springs up it's tough to put it back in the box. Jobs are good. We depend on jobs, yet, statistically speaking in a covariant sort of way, the difference in the incidence of heart disease between Finland and Greece could as easily have been correlated positively to Lapland reindeer or negatively to Mediterranean sponges.

Epidemiological studies more reliably indicate differences between populations than attribute causes to those differences. There were simply too many contributing dietary variables for conclusions to be drawn from the Seven Countries Study, but nobody knew that, because nothing like this had ever been done before.

Dr. Keys became famous and was featured on a 1961 cover of Time magazine. The media had cholesterol, saturated fats, and the devil all walking side-by-side en route to the morgue, and it was inevitable that studies seemingly linking dietary fat and heart disease would lead to studies of the effects of fat on cancer.

This work took two general forms. First, laboratory experiments measured the relative effects of various quantities and kinds of fat on the initiation and growth of tumors in rats and mice; and second, epidemiological studies compared cancer rates in various populations of humans with the amounts of fat they ate.

The cumulative data from early experiments on rats and mice certainly seemed to connect dietary fat with cancer. A 1975 summary of these findings concluded that both lower overall calories and lower overall fat limited cancer development, and that beneficial effects were most apparent in the early stages of disease, when the individual cells appeared relatively more susceptible to external influences.

For instance, in one experiment, fifty-one mice were fed a potent carcinogen. Thirty-two of the mice ate a normal mixed diet, and all thirty-two mice developed tumors. Nineteen of the mice were fed a low calorie diet in which carbohydrates and fats were cut in half; three of the mice developed tumors. In several similar experiments control groups of mice had cancer incidence rates of 40-67 percent, while groups of mice fed diets restricted in total calories by 50-75 percent had cancer incidence rates of 0-2 percent.

Kind of makes you want to push your plate away, doesn't it?

The effects of dietary fat, like total caloric intake, appeared to most affect cancers in their early stages, and had a dramatic effect on whether or not human breast cancer cells transplanted into mice grew into full blown tumors. In one experiment, 6 percent of mice fed a diet containing less than 0.5 percent lard developed mammary tumors, while 78 percent of mice fed a diet containing more than 15 percent lard developed tumors, demonstrating beyond a reasonable doubt that if you're a lard-eating female mouse on a diet of potent carcinogens you have cause for grave concern when it comes to breast cancer.

Rodents are used in these experiments because they're relatively cheap and easy to breed, because of the genetic and biological similarities between mice and men, and because you can do things to rodents you can't do to humans. One thing you can do to mice is breed out the thymus gland, an organ which is necessary to mount a standard immune response to implanted tissue. A side effect of not having a thymus gland is hair loss, and rather than calling them bald, these mice are described as "nude."

The results of laboratory experiments on nude mice must be applied with caution to women in little black dresses. Still, inferences can be drawn, and the premise that fat affects cancer in people was supported by some epidemiological studies that apparently showed statistically significant correlations between dietary fat intake and the incidence of breast, prostate, and intestinal cancers in human populations.

One particularly influential 1975 paper correlated food balance sheets with breast cancer rates in over one hundred countries, and found a very strong link between total dietary fat intake and breast cancer rates. In fact, between third world countries such as Thailand, where people ate about two ounces of total fat a day, and first world countries such as the Netherlands, where people ate about five ounces, this study found a five- to tenfold difference in age adjusted mortality rates from human breast cancer.

A tenfold difference is 1,000 percent. It's a colossal number, and when you consider that the benefits of most treatments are measured in tens of percent, it gives you some of idea of the magnitude of the potential health benefits of dietary changes.

Something powerful is going on, but what?

This study also found a very high correlation between the intake of animal fats and breast cancer, but no relationship whatsoever between the intake of vegetable fats and breast cancer. Therefore, the five- to tenfold differences in breast cancer rates are probably associated with the animals we eat, but probably not with the vegetables we eat. One—but far from the only—difference between animals and vegetables is that animals contain a higher proportion of saturated fats, and it was this difference upon which both the scientific community and the media pounced.

By the mid 1970s it had been "proven" that cholesterol causes heart disease and saturated fats cause breast cancer. The twin evils of saturated fats and cholesterol became a runaway publicity train full of cash cows. This train was roaring down the tracks, even though the emperor it carried wore no clothes.

A 1981 book reviewing the literature on diet, cholesterol, and heart disease accused Ancel Keys in his Seven Countries Study of cherry picking countries that upheld his theories and leaving out countries that didn't. His methodology was deemed inconsistent, his data rife with contradictions, which was what you'd expect of a study conducted with such scientific abandon. It was dumbfounding that rave reviewers ignored such sloppiness, inconceivable that objective scientists would take this work seriously.

That's some high powered scientific sniping.

The emperor has no clothes.

In the fable, the emperor is naked, but, because he's emperor, everybody compliments his outfit. With cholesterol, the original premise that this molecule is responsible for coronary disease had been shown to be without scientific basis, yet research continued as if cholesterol caused coronary disease. Adding to the irony, the once revered Doctor Keys was increasingly vilified in the scientific community.

Researchers discredited Keys, yet they kept his false premise.

For three reasons, I think they got it exactly backwards.

First, Doctor Keys placed emphasis on cholesterol, but only in the context of a larger dietary whole. Second, the Seven Countries Study didn't prove cholesterol causes heart disease, but it sure as hell showed that something does, and Keys attributed this less to cholesterol and more to "the North American habit of making the stomach a garbage disposal for a long list of harmful foods." Third, by following his own advice to eat a Mediterranean-like diet rich in olive oil, whole grains, beans, and vegetables along with a little meat, Keys lived to be two months shy of his hundredth birthday.

There's more of that anecdotal evidence.

With the Seven Countries Study, for the first time it had been shown different populations with different diets had vastly different rates of disease, and the first time for anything is a learning experience. Plus, if you design an experiment to test the effect of cholesterol on heart disease, you tend to find that effect. It's just how scientific reductionism works. Plus, to greater and lesser extents, every scientist cherry picks data prior to massaging it with a fudge factor. It's not cheating, really; it's just that science is imprecise and results are important, at least if you want continued funding.

Science has been jumping to conclusions for centuries. The epidemiological truth can almost never be boiled down to a single variable yet we keep trying, and, as for picking what variables to study...come on all you really smart science guys.

Saturated fatty acids keep us solid at room temperature, while cholesterol is a fundamental difference between the membranes of plant and animal cells. These molecules, as much as anything, make human cells possible. They're not bad for us, they're essential to us, and the idea that molecules we can't live without would be the root cause behind some of the worst diseases known to mankind must be causing Doctor Spock to roll over in his Vulcan grave.

"But captain...that is simply...illogical."

A breast is (among other wonderful things) a particularly shapely arrangement of saturated fatty acids, and the premise that saturated fats are bad for breasts makes as much sense as saying wood is bad for trees. Still, something must be causing that tenfold difference in breast cancer rates between countries that eat two ounces of fat a day as opposed to five ounces of fat a day, which brings us to the Nurses' Health Study, an ongoing epidemiological project generally considered to be among the best of its kind.

This study began in 1976 with 121,700 women aged 30-55, who were enrolled to evaluate how long term use of a popular new drug, the oral contraceptive, would affect breast cancer. The original cohort (study group) consisted of married women because in those archaic times you couldn't get a prescription for the pill unless you lived in a state of holy matrimony; the cohort consisted entirely of nurses based on the assumption that medical professionals would have a broad based knowledge of health issues and therefore their self-reported data would be more trustworthy.

Initially, every two years the enrolled nurses were asked to fill out a simple questionnaire on their habits, including smoking and hair dye use, but the study has evolved into a much more complicated phenomenon over time. A dietary questionnaire was included in 1980, and over 60,000 toenail samples were collected in 1983 to assess selenium levels. A second cohort was selected in 1989 and 33,000 blood samples were collected. The questionnaire became increasingly detailed through the years, more blood and then urine samples were collected, and in the year 2000, 35,000 DNA samples were collected and stored.

The study is considered to be notable for the high degree of follow-up among participants (over 90 percent), the collection of biological samples, and the overall low cost for follow-up, which as of 2005 was approximately fourteen dollars per participant per year. Crunch the numbers and, as of 2007, you come up with a total cost of nearly ninety million dollars, which also goes to show that it's good work if you can get it.

A lot of it *is* good work.

For instance, analyses based on Nurses' Health Study data have shown that seven or more hours of exercise per week reduces the risk of breast cancer by 20 percent and the risk of colon cancer by 40 percent. Other research has linked a high body-mass index (weight in kilograms divided by height in meters squared) to breast cancer. This, to me, seems like self-reported data you can trust. The nurses either exercise an hour a day or they don't. Their height and weight are their height and weight. It's black and white.

Self-reported dietary intake is a much grayer area. I don't believe nurses would intentionally lie about what they ate, but in the age of industrially processed foods, unless you run every bite through a mass spectrometer, there is no telling what you just ate. Garbage in, garbage out. It's as true of science as it is of your body, and this factor must be considered when divining the results of one of the largest epidemiological cancer studies in the history of the solar system, a widely cited 1996 study that pooled data from large studies in Sweden, the Netherlands, Canada, the states of California, Iowa, and New York, and the Nurses' Health Study.

In all, data was examined from 337,819 women, who reported 4,980 cases of breast cancer. The incidence of breast cancer was adjusted for risk factors such as body-mass index and family history; the adjusted numbers were then compared to dietary levels of total fat, saturated fat, unsaturated fat, animal fat, vegetable fat, and cholesterol. To calculate relative risk researchers then "exponentiated the appropriate conditional logistic-regression coefficient multiplied by a nutritionally meaningful increment for continuous variables."

The exponentiation of meaningful conditionals describes the fudge factor of choice, and after a tremendous amount of data manipulation, no statistically significant relationship was found between the dietary intake of any of the studied fats and breast cancer. The study found an equal risk of breast cancer in women who ate less than 25 percent of their energy as fat and nurses who ate more than 45 percent of their energy from fat, and concluded that, "in the context of the western lifestyle, lowering the total intake of fat in midlife is unlikely to reduce the risk of breast cancer substantially."

Another day, another epidemiological all-or-nothing medical flip-flop.

In the world of scientific either-or, where this study had a large impact, the conventional wisdom was now that there was "no evidence of a positive association between total dietary fat intake and the risk of breast cancer." The results were often described as "surprising" because there was so much evidence that fats did in some way affect breast cancer, and I can think of at least one reason for that surprise.

No accounting was made for trans fats in this huge epidemiological study, even though the dietary data was collected between 1977 and 1992, years when the use of partially hydrogenated oils was booming. In those days trans fats were our friends, saturated fats the foe. Artificial oils increasingly filled the deep fat fryers of our restaurants, while a host of svelte new products were created to satisfy the marketing niche created by the burgeoning new "low fat" food industry.

Health conscious nurses switching away from foods high in saturated fats to foods low in saturated fats, under the informational imperatives of the time, would also have been switching toward a higher intake of trans fats. Go to the store in the 1980s and stock up on low fat salad dressing, low fat crackers, low fat this, and low fat that, and you would report yourself as eating a low fat diet, although levels of trans fat would likely be high, a factor that could potentially mask the overall data on the effects of low versus high fat diets on cancer.

As evidence, consider a 2007 study that examined the levels of trans fats in blood samples taken from women participating in the Nurses' Health Study in 1989 and 1990. The 495 women selected showed that an average of 1.69 percent of the total fatty acids in their red blood cells were trans fats, and group levels ranged from 1.17 percent to 2.23 percent. These nurses could easily have reported themselves as eating healthy diets, yet at nearly 2 percent plastic in their cells, they were instead well on the way to ushering in the age of robotics.

This study also linked each incremental 0.25 percent increase in trans fats levels to a rise in adjusted relative coronary risk of about 30 percent. This corresponds to an average of 200 percent increased coronary risk in the study group, which could easily mask the effects of other risk factors. Epidemiological studies will always be better at determining effect rather than singling out cause, in part because there is no one single cause.

After decades of research, there's no compelling evidence that any one natural fatty acid is particularly bad for you. On the other hand, on many medical fronts, there is good evidence that limiting the calories you eat, in part by limiting the calorie-rich fats you eat, reduces your risk factors for many diseases, including the big three of atherosclerosis, type-2 diabetes, and cancer, by tens, hundreds, and perhaps thousands of percent.

Again, these are numbers you want on your side.

Even if all you do is avoid the trans fats hidden in processed foods, which will in turn help you avoid the calories typical of processed foods, then you've already taken two giant steps toward better cellular health. As for other dietary changes you might wish to make if you're truly serious about fighting or avoiding cancer, it seems the nurses' data might hold another clue.

The Nurses' Health Study has a 97 percent correlation with overall American breast cancer rates, and breast cancer rates in the United States are as much as ten times higher than in other countries with very different diets. Whatever Americans do that increases the chance of getting breast cancer, the nurses are likely to be doing it too, and as it turns out nurses are by nature a particularly carnivorous lot.

American nurses eat a lot of meat by any standards except for maybe those of wolves. The human RDA government recommended intake of protein (0.8 grams per 2.2 pounds of body weight) works out for me to about 10 percent of daily calories, while the typical American gets 15-16 percent, and 70 percent of that protein comes from animal sources. Nurses make good money and reported that they get about 19 percent of their calories from protein, of which 78-86 percent comes from relatively expensive animal sources.

Compare this with rural areas of China, where breast cancer rates are extremely low, and a mere 10 percent of the day's protein comes from animal sources. There's an obvious correlation between saturated fats and cholesterol and animal protein because the associated molecules are concentrated in the same flesh. Could there be a link between animal protein and cancer that was originally attributed to saturated fats?

If so, I wasn't so sure I wanted to know about it.

Me, I like meat.

But worse, I love cheese.

The Quadruple Whammy

W hen I was in the throes of treatment I had no idea how much lifestyle changes might affect my survival chances. My doctors didn't tell me and I didn't have time to find out. If I only had two years to live then I was going to live it up. I was barbequing every night. The idea that I could eat too much protein for my own good simply never occurred to me, and probably wouldn't have, not in a thousand years.

More dogma.

The first inkling that I might have been misinformed came when I read a book called *The China Study* by Joseph Campbell, who as a child was raised on a dairy farm. His father or one of the neighbors could have been the man who showed up in Ancel Key's laboratory with lumps of cholesterol over his eyebrows. Young Joseph was raised according to the holy trinity of beef, butter, and cheese, and later became a scientist, at which time the now Doctor Campbell became involved in researching the causes of extremely high rates of liver cancer in children in the Philippines in the 1960s.

Liver cancer generally strikes people late in life, but Filipino children were dying as young as four years old. Aflatoxin, an extremely potent carcinogen, had recently been discovered to thrive in a mold that grows on peanuts. In the Philippines, good peanuts were going into tins for export as fancy mixed nuts; moldy peanuts were going into the local peanut butter, and the peanut butter was going into the kids.

A steady diet of aflatoxin was reasoned to be the cause of a high incidence of liver cancer in Filipino children younger than ten years old but, oddly, only the rich kids were dying of liver cancer. The poor kids ate the same peanut butter, but they weren't developing liver cancer. Filipino poverty can be extreme, and you'd think it would be the other way around, that poor kids with poor diets would be more susceptible to liver cancer as they are more susceptible to other illnesses.

This anomaly was investigated by scientists in India, who eventually published in an obscure journal their results on the combined effects of protein and aflatoxin on liver cancer in laboratory rats. The experiment was simple. Two groups of rats were exposed to equivalent amounts of aflatoxin; then one group was fed a diet that included 20 percent protein, while the other group was fed a diet containing only 5 percent protein. Every rat fed the high protein diet developed cancer or precancerous lesions; none of the rats fed the low protein diet developed cancer or lesions.

All the rats had problems, or none of the rats had problems.

In science, results like this are unheard of. It just doesn't happen that it's 100 percent one way, and 100 percent the other way, so the results were easily dismissed. Perhaps the dead rats had inadvertently been slipped some poison. At any rate something went wrong. The data was flawed. Nobody wanted to hear that the sacred cow of protein was bad for you, but Doctor Campbell, having observed firsthand the horrors of liver cancer in the Filipino children, pursued the investigation.

Doctor Campbell, a shrewd political operator, realized that grant money was unlikely to be forthcoming for an experiment specifically designed to investigate proteins as potential carcinogens. Protein was then and is now a food-pyramid captain of the government-sponsored home team. In that game the home team always gets the calls, so Campbell's original grant was written to examine the effects of "various factors" on the development of liver cancer in rodents.

Plus, it was good science to check out other factors, and in the investigation of the various substances potentially promoting cancer, the effects of protein appeared time and time again. From initiation through growth and into metastasis, the influence of protein on cancer proved to be fertile ground for research—the results compelling enough that Doctor Campbell managed to acquire funding for twenty-seven more years of experiments.

The initiation of cancer can begin when a carcinogen such as aflatoxin enters a cell, and is acted upon by enzymes to produce a more reactive chemical, a chemical that then attaches tightly to cellular DNA, forming an *adduct.* If this now damaged cell reproduces before the genetic damage can be repaired, perhaps because you haven't been eating your carrots and your repair crews are short of the supplies found concentrated in carrots, then the cancer is said to have initiated.

Experiments on mice showed that low protein diets first lowered the amount of aflatoxin that entered the cell, and then diminished the enzyme activity necessary to build the DNA-attacking adducts. Surprisingly, it had been shown that protein directly affected the initiation of cancer at two different way stations in the Pony Express system of chemical messengers, results that led to further research.

If initiation is the seed of cancer, then promotion is the sprouting. Promotion begins with the growth of a cluster of cancer-like cells called *foci,* and foci development was found to be almost entirely dependent on protein intake, as opposed to carcinogen exposure. In other words, liver cancer almost always sprouted in rats on a high protein diet, while cancer almost never sprouted in rats on a low protein diet, independent of how much aflatoxin the rats were being fed.

More experiments showed that foci growth could be manipulated, at all stages, according to levels of protein intake. Up, down, and all around, protein made the cancer dance. Low protein intake appeared to make existing tumors shrink; high protein intake caused an increase in a growth hormone that both fed the tumor like fertilizer and encouraged cancer cells to break free and colonize. To find even one link between dietary protein and the initiation, growth, and metastasis of cancer would have been interesting; to find it at so many levels in all three stages was compelling.

The mice were certainly convinced.

Immunity-impaired nude mice are unable to defend against foreign tissue. They can therefore be implanted with various cancers, and the growth of living tumors can then be measured in response to the manipulated factor of choice, including dietary protein levels. In mice, sprouting of the initial cancer seed increased rapidly at levels above 10 percent dietary protein levels. It is probably no coincidence that both rodents and humans seem to require a ballpark average of about 10 percent of their daily calories as protein for normal growth and maintenance.

Data from nude mice does not strictly apply to humans, nude or otherwise. Still, it would be folly to chalk up so much evidence on so many levels to coincidence. This progression of experiments culminated in a study of hundreds of rats over a hundred-week period meant to approximate the typical two-year rat lifespan, and the ingestion of protein was shown to affect the development of cancer in many ways.

As one example, rats switched from high to low protein diets during the study showed 35-40 percent less tumor growth. In the most telling example, at the end of a hundred weeks all the afla-toxin-infected rats on a 20 percent protein diet were dead or near dead from liver tumors; all the rats on a 5 percent protein diet were alive and thriving.

That's not just some, that's all.

To me, that's astonishing.

The protein used in these studies was casein, the main protein in cow's milk.

Earlier epidemiological studies on humans had shown breast cancer seemed to be linked to animal but not vegetable fats, so the question became whether animal protein and vegetable protein had different effects on liver tumor development. As an example of what researchers found, in one experiment on cancer growth, rats fed diets of 20 percent soy protein or 20 percent gluten (wheat protein) did not demonstrate high levels of early foci development, while rats on a 20 percent casein diet did. It seemed that it wasn't just any protein that promoted cancer growth; it was animal-based protein.

How could this be?

How could meat be bad for you?

I mean, look at Lewis and Clark. Those guys hunted their way across the United States back when the hunting was good. A lot of those elk, deer, buffalo, ducks, rabbits, and grouse were seeing guns for the first time. The men in that expedition ate several pounds of meat a day, day in and day out, for nearly three years, yet only one man died.

Part of the answer must lie in the difference between dragging a boat upstream for a thousand miles and sitting at your desk with your belly hanging over your belt. It's a huge difference in how much protein the body needs to replenish itself. Too much saturated fat is like too much animal protein is like too much of anything. The body can't keep up. It's an overdose. All those extra molecules have to go somewhere, and when they do, balances are upset.

It's like you have a one-bedroom apartment and ten relatives show up. You can get by for a while with people sleeping on the couch and under the kitchen table, but before long you have kissing cousins and inbred children on the fire escape playing the theme from *Deliverance* on the banjo. Mutations can arise in crowded cells and crowded houses because too much of anything means something has to give, and, when it comes to prostate cancer, it seems dairy products give and then give some more.

A 2001 Harvard review of the research, based on positive associations in nineteen out of twenty-three different studies, concluded consumption of dairy products is "one of the most consistent dietary predictors for prostate cancer in the published literature." The study estimated that high dairy intake more than doubled the risk of developing prostate cancer, and about quadrupled the risk of developing fatal prostate cancer, and one reason this might be true involves the chemical vitamin D.

Vitamins are organic compounds essential to diverse bodily processes. Some vitamins are soluble in water, and some, like steroids, are soluble in fat. Vitamins are complex molecules, generally constructed by plants, using the direct energy of the sun. Humans can't generally make these high energy molecules, but fat-soluble vitamin D, a bent chain containing both rings and strings of carbon, is the exception to the rule.

Get enough sun and specialized skin cells spit out all the vitamin D you need. The manufactured vitamin D is then transported through the blood and stored mostly in the liver as a fairly stable metabolite, molecules which we'll call storage D, stored molecules that are available at a moment's notice.

Storage D, when called for by chemical signals from the parathyroid, rides the blood from the liver to the kidneys, where it is processed within seconds into molecules of a new and highly reactive nature we'll simply call active D. Active D does the actual work in your cells, and that vitamin D stores messages in one place in your body and processes them in another is just one tiny example of the sophisticated and intricate elegance of the checks and balances that drive your chemical messaging system.

Molecules of active D are a thousand times more reactive than molecules of storage D, and molecules of active D tend to exist for about six to eight hours, as opposed to twenty days or more for storage D. Short-lived active D adjusts within seconds to change, long-lived storage D provides the ready supplies that make these quick changes possible, and the whole system tends back to neutral over a matter of hours.

If only my checkbook were always so balanced.

Right now, there are kids out there saying, "What's a checkbook?"

Life is change.

Vitamin D assists enzymes in essential chemical reactions specific to different cells, and chronically low levels of active D are associated with diseases as diverse as cancer, osteoporosis, and multiple sclerosis. Active D is an influential metabolite, and casein in the blood creates an acidic environment that interferes with the enzyme activity that leads to active D. It's chemistry. An animal-protein-rich, acidic environment stalls production of active D, and low levels of active D are in turn strongly linked to high rates of prostate cancer.

But wait, there's more...

This is like one of those infomercials for knives.

If you call in the next five minutes...

Dairy products that tend to be high in the animal protein casein also tend to be high in calcium. High levels of calcium in the blood cause active D to become less active, and active D levels are already low because of casein-induced acidic blood. It's a double whammy. Active D is getting hit from the front and the flank.

But wait, there's more.

And it's even worse.

Insulin-like growth factor 1 (IGF-1) is a naturally produced human protein that triggers cell growth and reproduction. Increased levels of IGF-1 in laboratory animals have been shown to increase rates of cancer cell reproduction, to inhibit the ordinary reaction of mutated cells to destroy themselves, and to encourage mutated cells to spread. This is not a chemical with which you want your cancer cells to tinker; yet, diets high in animal protein have been shown to chemically stimulate levels of IGF-1 in mice, and studies on humans have shown that men with higher than normal levels of IGF-1 have over five times the risk of advanced-stage prostate cancer.

But wait, there's more.

Trans fatty acids are rare in nature, with the notable exception of ruminants, such as cows. Ruminants have rumens, an extra stomach containing specialized bacteria able to break down the cellulose in the grasses ruminants eat. These specialized bacteria churn out some trans fats as a normal part of the digestion of cellulose, enough that trans fats comprise roughly 4-6 percent of the total fats in ruminant meat and dairy products. The jury is still out on whether these naturally produced trans fats are as bad for you as industrially produced trans fats, but this much is certain:

Bite for bite, as compared to almost any other food you might choose to eat, the particular blend of molecules characteristic of dairy products results in more trans fats, more insulin-like growth factor, less active D, and more overall calories.

This all amounts to a quadruple whammy of high powered cancer risk factors, which, sadly, make me a statistic. I figure I've eaten two or three tons of cheese over the course of my lifetime, and my prostate ended up riddled with high grade cancer, just as a high consumption of dairy products would predict.

What's funny...ha, ha, ha...is how I thought I had a pretty healthy diet.

I knew because it said so on the back of the box.

Silly me.

Sorry Guys, Size Matters

Nobody can tell you exactly what to eat because we're as different on the inside as we are on the outside. Just because a bikini looks good on a supermodel doesn't mean it will look good on you, and just because your neighbor eats tofu doesn't mean you should too.

I tried being a vegetarian and it didn't suit me. At the same time, too much meat makes my cells want to lie down and take a nap. If a food is to fight cancer it must work at the cellular level, and, as far as our cells are concerned, the matter can be boiled down to three kinds of food.

First, there is the food we should never eat, second, there is the food we must eat, and third, there is everything else.

The food we should never eat isn't really food, it's just found in food, and includes trans fats, the chemical derivatives of mercury, the neurotoxins in insecticides, preservatives, and on and on. Some of these substances are harder on your cells than others, and effects are cumulative, so the more you eat of these chemicals the worse it is.

The food we have to eat includes all the chemicals our cells need but can't make for themselves. These include minerals such as iron, vitamins, polyunsaturated fatty acids, several amino acids, water, and oxygen.

Then, there's everything else.

This is the food that supplies the bulk of the raw materials and energy sources your cells need to keep you alive. It is just as essential to your health as the food you have to eat, and there are no magic bullets. You don't just need some of these things, you need them all, and too much of any one thing can be just as bad as too little.

It's like you're framing a house. You'll need two-by-fours for the interior walls, two-by-sixes for the exterior walls, and two-by-tens for floor joists and rafters. You'll need all those pieces in different lengths, and it's a lot easier if the wood is delivered in the sizes you want at the time you need it. Otherwise you have to move everything around before you can get anything done. It's make-work.

You can build a house out of raw trees but it's way harder. It takes energy and time to make the right pieces out of the wrong pieces, and creates waste, which has to go somewhere. You might even wear out a table saw ripping the large pieces down to size, and when you finally get the right pieces, you still have to put them together.

It isn't an efficient way of doing business. If you were a contractor you couldn't compete with a competitor who had parts delivered pre-made. It's the same with the manufacturing plants that are our cells, and the more highly processed a food is, the less likely it is to have what you need, and the more likely it is to have what you don't need.

As an example of how even the best of foods can turn on you, consider the essential omega-3 linolenic and omega-6 linoleic fatty acids, molecules with high energy bonds our cells are incapable of manufacturing. Conventional wisdom holds that we should eat as much of these "good" fatty acids as we can, yet many studies show that the relative balance between these fatty acids is a more reliable indicator of health.

This is in part because omega-6 linoleic acid is the precursor to a molecule that stimulates inflammation, while omega-3 linolenic acid is the precursor to a slightly different molecule that triggers the anti-inflammatory response. Too much on and not enough off can lead to chronic inflammation, and the temperatures characteristic of industrial food processing tend to destroy more omega-3 fatty acids than omega-6 fatty acids. Crank up omega-6 levels by munching almost any processed food you care to mention, and you're also cranking up the on-switch to chronic inflammation.

But wait, there's more.

We don't think of steak as being processed like a breakfast pastry, but cows, like people, are what they eat. Omega-3 linolenic acid is a major component in many pasture grasses and free-range beef. Cows processed in the feed lot, however, are fattened on omega-6-rich corn. Omega-6 fatty acids preferentially replace the omega-3 acids, and if you eat feed lot beef, you're also cranking up the inflammatory on-switch.

Inflammation is a basic immune response that is not meant to be maintained indefinitely. Chronic inflammation is no better for you than chronic stress, and while a ballpark estimate of the proper ratio of omega-6 to omega-3 is two-to-one, actual ratios in typical diets are more like ten- to thirty-to-one. The result is an imbalance in the direction of chronic inflammation, which is exacerbated by eating processed oils rich in polyunsaturated fatty acids, even though these are advertised as the healthiest of oils.

Too much fat, too much protein, too much food, too much of anything is too much for you. Every bite you eat goes through several levels of processing. Extra food requires extra work, which requires extra energy, and if a cell lacks that, energy systems begin to go awry. Plus, extra work means extra waste. Every calorie you eat has to go somewhere, and it doesn't take much of a frozen pizza habit before you become the cellular equivalent of buzzards circling Mount Trashmore.

Remember the old *I Love Lucy* television show?

There's Lucy, taking pies off a conveyor belt, putting them in boxes, neatly piling them for delivery. Cherry pies go in the red boxes, apple pies in the green. Then, the conveyor belt speeds up. As pies come faster they're packaged in the wrong boxes. Lucy's getting behind, she starts eating pies as they go by. The conveyor belt speeds up again. No way can Lucy handle the barrage and the system breaks down. It's pies in her blouse, pies in her pants, pies kicked to the side, until finally the boss shows up.

"Lucy...you're fired."

"Cells...you're mutated."

It's not that animal foods are inherently bad for us; it's just that high levels of certain nutrients in animal foods add up in a hurry. We're very good at making most of these molecules for ourselves, but they still taste good. So, anticancer animal-food-wise, how much is too much?

As a ballpark dietary guideline, consider limiting animal protein intake to about 10 percent of your daily calories, and total fat intake to about 20 percent of your daily calories. It might not be a diet you'd care to eat on a daily basis, but, then again, especially if you're fighting a tumor, it might.

As a matter of reference, 10 percent of a 2000-calorie-a-day diet in animal protein works out to about eight ounces of cheddar cheese, or eight ounces of ground beef, seven ounces of lean chicken, ten ounces of salmon, or seven cups of milk. In those same portions the cheese would give you about 35 percent of your total daily calories of fat; beef, 18 percent; chicken, 4 percent; and milk, 25 percent of total daily calories as fat in a typical 2000-calorie-a-day diet. If you want to eat more fat don't cut back on nutrient-rich carbohydrates, get more exercise.

Burn, baby, burn.

In any given day call it a mix-and-match of an ounce or two of cheese, a quarter pound of meat, and a glass of milk. If you're serious about a low fat diet, consider that a tablespoon of any cooking oil contains 120 calories, and three tablespoons of oil gives you about 18 percent of your daily calories as fat even if you don't eat any meat or cheese.

It's not much, but then that's the whole point. It was different than what I'd been doing, and different was good. This was something I could change, so I did.

I'm no vegan.

But color me increasingly natural.

The problem with processed foods is twofold. First, they're rich in molecules we should never eat. Second, processing concentrates quantities of some molecules, while destroying others, and the molecules that are most easily destroyed are the ones we can't make, like vitamins and polyunsaturated fatty acids.

As an example of how processing can be detrimental to your cells, consider palm oil, now the world's largest commodity traded food oil. Palm oil is highly processed, and steps typically include refining, bleaching, deodorizing, and fractionation into liquid and solid components before sale as a variety of end products.

The liquid fraction of palm oil contains a lower proportion of saturated fats, and is used in everything from cosmetics to energy production. The solid component created by fractionation, palm butter, contains a high proportion of saturated fats, is pervasive in processed baked goods, and contains very few of the essential molecules you must eat and far more of a few saturated fatty acids than you can use. The discarded component of the original oil includes a rich red stream of beta carotene, essential antioxidants your cells crave, that instead ends up on the jungle floor.

You can eat fractionated palm butter until you're the size of a blimp and still be missing a whole sheaf of essential nutrients. If you are missing these nutrients, and you then supply them, then your cells will function better, perhaps greatly so. It is easy to see how this can help prevent cells from becoming cancerous, but what about the effect of dietary changes on cancer cells that are already there?

Can you eat your way out of a tumor?

Or maybe at least snack on it?

Molecular Miracles

Cancer involves cellular energy deficits, and, if cellular energy deficits are involved, then so is the plasma cell membrane. Depending on who you talk to, the membrane that separates the energy inside the cell from the energy outside the cell is either a miracle or a marvel of bioengineering. The Pope would steer you one way, Darwin another, and maybe they're both right because the molecules that form the fabric of the membrane are nothing if not a study in contrasts.

These linear molecules are polar at one end, and nonpolar at the other. In the presence of water these molecules form up like a marching band, their polar heads always pointing toward polar water. The fatty nonpolar feet are in turn attracted to the fatty nonpolar feet of another marching band, creating a bi-layer of mirror image molecular marching bands that don't like to get their fat feet wet.

The polar heads of these mirror image marching bands point out, the nonpolar feet point in, and as the bands get bigger the same forces that cause oil to form droplets in water cause the membrane to fold back upon itself into a bubble. The film on that bubble is the miracle of life, and it's a marvel because the electrical imperatives of the universe are satisfied, all in a membrane that's only two molecules thick.

The polar heads both give and receive water-based messages, while the inner layer of dual fats isolates the contents of the cell both chemically and electrically from the world at large. Without this bi-layer of fats you'd go up in sparks, like that time you dumped coffee in your keyboard, and it is the electrochemical potential across the plasma cell membrane that drives the force of life.

Electrical differences cause oxygen and other raw materials to enter the cell; electrical differences allow finished products like messenger proteins to leave. There's waste to get rid of, sometimes less, or, depending on your will power, sometimes more. The flow of molecules across the membrane is strictly controlled, and two molecules that are crucial to this electrochemical control are phospholipids and cholesterol.

Both of these molecules are members of the marching band with polar heads and nonpolar feet, but phospholipids are more linear because they're built around carbon chains, while cholesterol is more planar because it's built around carbon rings. Again, to use the house building analogy in your cell membrane, phospholipids would be like linear two-by-fours while cholesterol would be like planar plywood.

Frame up a wall with nothing but two-by-fours and you can collapse it with one hand, but once you sheathe it with plywood you can ram it with a truck if you don't mind hurting the truck. The difference is shear strength, and it isn't something cells really needed until they began to move around in mass quantities.

As animals we move, and cholesterol is a big reason our cells move with us. Plants don't have cholesterol, because they don't need it. Cholesterol is as fundamental to our animal nature as molecules come, so you can see why drugs that interfere with how our cells build and use this molecule have unintended consequences.

Phospholipids are a variation on the diglyceride theme, with two dangling nonpolar fatty acid legs. These legs can be straight saturated fatty acids, slightly bent monounsaturated fatty acids, or highly bent polyunsaturated acids. Phospholipids with straight legs pack more closely together, which decreases membrane permeability. Phospholipids with bent legs kick each other apart, which increases membrane permeability, and varying the ratio of these fatty acid legs in cell membranes is part of what gives different tissues different properties.

Now suppose you're a brain cell.

As a brain cell, you require a lot of oxygen, and the passage of that oxygen is facilitated by the high percentage of highly bent polyunsaturated fatty acids in your membrane. Next, suppose you're thinking really hard about what you're going to do with all that money once you win the lottery. Just the thought of it is so exciting you're gasping for breath. You need more oxygen, so you reach out for more highly-bent unsaturated fatty acids, but there aren't any.

You make do with a slightly bent fatty acid, but it's not the same. You're a little tired.

Or worse, maybe the mouth that feeds you just ate flour tortillas.

There's a reason white tortillas can sit in the refrigerator for weeks without turning green. You're a brain cell, you should know this. The nutrition facts label says zero grams trans fat, but the fine print says shortening, and your cell incorporates a straight leg where it was expecting a highly bent leg. Either way, from a lack of the right parts or an abundance of really wrong parts, the more you eat the worse the oxygen deficit gets.

Now suppose you're a cancer cell.

Phospholipids

It is a vast and improbable collection of molecules that together weave the tapestry of life. Human beings are the culmination of a pyramid of chemical innovations that have been conserved over time, and at the beating heart of the plasma cell membrane that defines all the life that follows are clever constructs of organic chemistry called phospholipids.

Phospholipids are both attracted to water, and repelled by water, because they combine the polar properties of proteins with the nonpolar properties of fats. Phosphatidylcholine, shown below, the most common phospholipid in human cell membranes, has a nonpolar end consisting of two fatty acids, and a polar end consisting of a positively charged nitrogen based choline molecule and a negatively charged phosphate group.

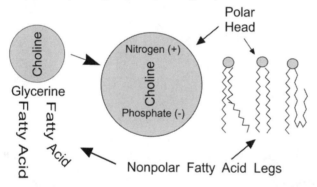

Fatty acid legs can be saturated, monounsaturated, or poly-unsaturated; the fatty acid carbon chain will bend at each unsaturated double bond, and the shape of each fatty acid contributes specific properties to the cell membrane.

The polar heads of these molecules are also interchangeable, and the result of this mixing and matching of heads and legs is several different molecules that exhibit varying kinds of bipolar behavior. Your car can't run without the right parts and neither can your cell membranes. You don't just need some of these molecules, you need them all, because if your cell membranes aren't healthy, then neither are you.

Plasma Cell Membrane

The polar ends of cholesterol and phospholipids will always line up facing polar water, and can thus form a bi-layer with the nonpolar fatty acids sandwiched between the polar heads. This bi-layer is flexible, semipermeable, and allows the maintenance of a different chemical and energetic environment in the water inside the cell as opposed to the water outside the cell.

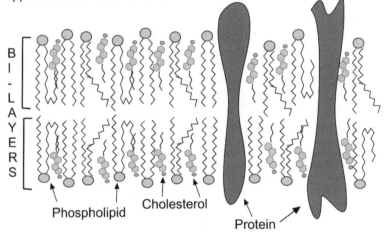

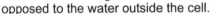

Phospholipid Cholesterol Protein

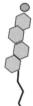 Cholesterol is found in all animal tissues in varying but substantial amounts, and generally comprises 30%-50% of the plasma membrane. The flat, rigid carbon ring structure of cholesterol modulates membrane fluidity through interactions with phospholipids, spans about half a bi-layer, fills in membrane gaps to decrease passive ionic diffusion, and can bond with the protein receptors and enzymes that span the bi-layer.

Messenger ligands (shown in black to right) arrive in the blood plasma, react with the receptor of a particular protein, creating an electrochemical message that is then transmitted through the protein and into the cell. Different cells have different proteins that respond to different chemical messengers, and the amount of protein in any given cell membrane can amount to as much as half of the total surface area.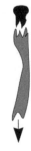

What if a bunch of the right parts came flooding in? What if the mouth that feeds you turned over a new leaf? What if there were no more trans fats to help plug up your cell membrane, and there was instead an abundance of high energy, highly bent, natural omega-3 fatty acids? Would that be enough to make you pull a Darth Vader?

Would that be enough to bring you back in from the dark side?

Would you go so far as to kill yourself for the common good?

In cells, ritual suicide is called *apoptosis,* and experiments on cell cultures, mice, and humans all show that omega-3 fatty acids do indeed encourage cancer cells to kill themselves. Omega-3 fatty acids have also been shown to interfere with the signaling pathways cancer uses, inhibit angiogenesis and significantly reduce overall proliferation of mutant cells. To find even one of these benefits would be promising, to find these fatty acids affect so many way stations in the Pony Express system of chemical messengers just means they are that much more likely to help.

The same high energy bonds that make omega-3 fatty acids good for us are also easily destroyed by heat, light, and oxygen. Omega-3 fatty acids don't travel well, but fortunately in at least one case they come with their own suitcase.

The suitcase is an oil-rich seed produced by the flowers of the flax plant, and inside that seed the oils are typically 10 percent saturated fats, 21 percent monounsaturated oleic acid, 16 percent omega-6 linoleic acid, and 53 percent omega-3 linolenic acid. Flaxseed oil is about the richest source of highly unsaturated fatty acids naturally available to us, and the high energy bonds in these fatty acids are protected by proportionately high quantities of a powerful antioxidant called lignin.

The levels of lignin in flax seed are typically seventy-five to eight hundred times those in other common dietary plant foods, and plant lignin is a precursor to mammalian lignin. Experiments have shown lignin interferes in many ways with the growth of tumors in laboratory mice, particularly in the processes involving cellular angiogenesis, proliferation, adhesion, migration, and invasion that characterize final metastasis.

Lignin affects some chemical pathways, highly unsaturated fatty acids affect several other chemical pathways, and together they're just that much more likely to interfere with the ability of cancer cells to grow and spread. High quality flax oil is generally cold-pressed and kept refrigerated to preserve the delicate bonds, and is a good example of the benefits of eating raw oil that comes with its nutritional integrity intact as opposed to oil in which the balance of nutrients has been processed out.

Early experiments showed a diet of 10 percent flax seed down-regulated production of two growth factors and impeded the receptors for a third growth factor in breast cancer cells implanted in mice. It's a big hurt on cancer to deprive it of the molecules that instruct it to grow, so a follow-up experiment was designed to examine the effects of the various components of flaxseed oil on the growth of live tumors.

The experiment began when cancerous human breast cells were injected into the breast pads of over one hundred live nude mice. The mice all lived on the same diet for the next eight weeks and showed similar tumor development, at which point the mice were separated into five groups. The first group continued to feed on the processed corn-oil-rich basal diet, the second on a diet that substituted 10 percent flax seed, the third on 10 percent flax oil, the fourth on 10 percent lignin, and the fifth on 10 percent flax oil plus lignin.

The mice were fed these various and strictly controlled diets for the next six weeks, at which time the mice were killed and their tumors autopsied. The total weight, volume, and palpability of the breast tumor were lower in all groups fed flax products as opposed to the control group. The incidence of metastasis into the lung was significantly decreased by 50 percent and 70 percent in the flax seed and oil plus lignin groups, and to lesser extents in the groups fed either oil or lignin but not both.

Our bodies are rife with redundant backup systems, and research indicates that just because cancer chemically overrides one line of apoptosis doesn't mean another line of apoptosis can't kick in later on. Cancer cells can come back from the dark side, and, significantly, in this study that is precisely what happened. The percentage of mutant cells that recognized systems were awry and triggered apoptosis increased in the flax seed, flax oil, and lignin plus oil groups by 65 percent, 60 percent, and 49 percent respectively.

That's a lot of dead cancer cells.

The study concluded that reduced primary tumor growth was due, in part, to reduced tumor cell proliferation and increased apoptosis. The study also concluded that oil and lignin together were more effective at inhibiting tumor metastasis effect than either oil or lignin individually, another example of the benefits of food that comes with all parts intact. It all amounts to several distinct lines of evidence that nutritionally intact flax seed beats back the initiation, growth, and particularly the metastasis of human breast cancer cells in test tubes and nude mice.

A 2005 Canadian study was designed to determine what, if any, effects flax seed might have on humans by first splitting thirty-two women with positive breast cancer biopsies into two groups. One group received a whole wheat muffin placebo, one group received a muffin in which 25 grams of ground flax seed replaced part of the wheat, and both groups continued the diet for a little over a month.

Daily food records were kept by the subjects, and no significant differences were found in total calorie and macronutrient intake other than the flax seed. The researchers were frank that the study sample was small and the results need confirmation, but they found the addition of dietary flax seed affected cancer in several hopeful ways.

Tumor cell proliferation decreased 34 percent, the index of apoptosis increased 31 percent, and the expression of a particularly unwelcome protein (C-erbB-2) associated with increased signaling between mutant cells and more aggressive tumors in a variety of cancers was decreased by a whopping 71 percent. Those are significant differences, but it's no more than what you would expect of molecules that can open the membrane by which cellular energy balances are kept to allow in more oxygen.

The Budwig Protocol

In a quote attributed to Albert Einstein, when attempting to solve a problem, "Everything should be made as simple as possible, but not simpler."

$E=mc^2$.

Energy is mass, and mass is energy.

Cancer is a disease of the cell, something has to cause it, and the idea that a simple lack of cellular energy might be responsible is both simple and elemental. For me, it was a whole new way of looking at how I might treat my cancer, but not at first.

At first it just seemed crazy.

At first, on Doctor Seed's advice I'd been eating flax oil, albeit on an irregular basis. I knew flax was rich in omega-3 oils, whatever they were, but not much more than that. I didn't know cellular energy deficits from budget deficits, and there I was, just another dumb guy with cancer, out in Southern California, doing my slide show for several fly-fishing clubs.

People at the premeeting pub-style dinners knew I had cancer because I'd written about it, and since attendees were mostly affluent male American baby-boomers, a particularly rich vein of troublesome prostates, it wasn't unusual for the conversation around the table to take a glandular turn.

"I had the surgery."

"Seeds for me."

"Chemotherapy…never again."

A guy in a Dodger's cap studded with trout flies hadn't had cancer, just an enlarged prostate that was closing down the tube draining his bladder.

"It's like trying to piss through a swizzle stick."

"I hope the neighbors weren't watching."

"What the hell happened? Do you remember when we used to sit at this table and talk about fishing instead of cholesterol?"

There was general agreement that nobody could be expected to remember that far back. Then, one night, I met a man named Chris. Chris, like me, had advanced prostate cancer, but unlike me, while he hadn't ruled out conventional treatments, he'd tried nonconventional treatments first, while keeping track of biomarkers that would indicate if his cancer were getting worse. Seven years later he'd never had to resort to conventional treatment, and his biomarkers, which he still had tested every three months, indicated he was essentially cancer free.

"So, what did you do?" I asked.

"The Budwig diet."

"The what?"

Johanna Budwig, a German biochemist, was nominated for seven Nobel Prizes in the years following World War II for her pioneering work in paper chromatography techniques that first allowed scientists to distinguish with precision between the various unsaturated fatty acids. Seven Nobel nominations is a good pedigree, and Chris was a bright-eyed disciple as he ticked off the high points in the anticancer gospel according to Budwig: minimize meat, fat, and processed foods; emphasize exposure to sunshine; and, crucially, add dietary flax oil in combination with cottage cheese.

Well, yeah, but...

"That's it?"

"It's enough..."

Chris went on to tell me how phosphorous-rich proteins in the cottage cheese combined with highly unsaturated fatty acids in the flax oil to form molecules called lipoproteins, which are easily digested and deliver the nutrients quickly and directly to cell membranes, which translated into immediate relief for the cells that needed these molecules most. This in turn restored normal cellular energy balances, which encouraged healthy cells to stay healthy and cancer cells to destroy themselves, and that was enough for Frau Budwig to use her protocol to save the lives of cancer patients so terminal they couldn't even swallow.

Well, yeah, but...

"If they couldn't swallow...how did they get their oil and cheese?"

"Enemas."

I'll say this for Chris, he didn't look like a wacko.

He looked good, slender, and vital, more like fifty than the sixty-five he gave as his age. He wasn't just alive, he was very much alive, at a time when the odds said he should have been long since dead. Whatever he'd done, it had worked.

On the other hand, when you get cancer, one side effect is well-meaning people briefing you on preposterous cures. For me, this included the recommendation that I eat nothing but mushrooms, on the theory that mushrooms are extraterrestrial in origin, because the spores were distributed by impacting comets, and fungi are therefore a foreign life form capable of destroying cancer cells.

At first, I found the idea that flax oil enemas might cure cancer to be only slightly less preposterous than the mushroom diet. Honestly, I was trying not to laugh, but Chris just smiled that beautiful smile people have when they've found peace with themselves.

"Check it out," he said.

So I did, and found that Frau Budwig, using her new experimental techniques to accurately measure the concentrations of the individual fatty acids, began examining the blood associated with the tumors of advanced cancer patients in the late 1940s. She described that blood as being first, oxygen deprived, and second, deficient in levels of phosphatides and lipoproteins containing highly unsaturated fatty acids. After many experiments Frau Budwig proposed a simple explanation for the fact that low levels of oxygen in cancerous blood were always associated with low levels of the omega-3 highly unsaturated fatty acids. Without adequate levels of these fatty acids, Doctor Budwig concluded from her work, "the enzymes in the breath cannot function, and we asphyxiate, even when given extra oxygen."

In other words, without these fatty acids we can't breathe.

That's pretty essential.

Our cells can't make these essential fatty acids because we don't have the chemistry to put unsaturated bonds at the third or sixth position up from the end of a fatty acid chain. Such high energy feats generally require the power of the sun, and the power of the sun is behind a host of other nutrients essential to our health that our cells can't make and we must get from the foods we eat. Without vitamin C, gums bleed and teeth rot with scurvy. Vitamin B1, or thiamine, prevents the nerve disorder beriberi, while a deficiency in vitamin B2 interferes with protein metabolism and causes cataracts. In similar fashion, according to Budwig, a deficiency in the essential fatty acids interferes with proper respiration and causes cancer.

Could it be that simple?

This was the very first time I'd heard cancer described in terms of energy, and the more I read the more sense it made. Ninety years of research definitively links cancer with cellular oxygen deficits and the chemical messengers created by those oxygen deficits, and Frau Budwig further proposed an elementary dietary solution to the problem as she defined it.

Since blood associated with tumors was consistently deficient in both essential fatty acids and phosphatides, she thought to restore the unsaturated fatty acids with flax oil, and the phosphatides with the proteins in cottage cheese. They didn't know then, but we do know now, that these are key ingredients in phosphatidylcholine, a major molecular player in the regulation of respiration in the cell membrane.

Doctor Budwig was on to something early on when she linked respiration with fatty acids, and for her continuum of work she was repeatedly nominated for the Nobel Prize. The Frau might have won one, even in what was very much a scientific old boy's club, if she'd stopped there. But she didn't. Frau Budwig was a scientific rabble-rouser, speaking out fiercely against, among other sacred cows, the flawed nature of radiation and chemotherapy as cancer treatments. According to her, the very worst way to fight cancer was to further weaken the cells.

You can imagine how that went over.

Doctor Budwig spoke vociferously against the use of DDT twenty years before the poison was finally banned, citing high cancer rates in populations of foresters and vintners, who were spraying insecticides on their trees and grapes respectively. Frau Budwig also attacked the food industry from her one-time position as German Senior Expert on Fats when, while investigating the effects of hydrogenated fish oils as fattening additives in animal feed cake, she observed that "50 percent of the pigs fatted on the (hydrogenated) feed cake turned blue and died on the way to the slaughterhouse."

The fatty acids in fish can have up to five unsaturated bonds. If you change all five bonds from cis bonds to trans bonds you have not just an unnatural molecule but an extremely unnatural molecule. Indeed, several studies show the detrimental effects of trans fats increase dramatically as the number of trans bonds in any given fatty molecule increases. This is a fine example of how cumulative effects are increasingly detrimental, because it is no small feat to turn half your pigs blue on the way to market.

Senior Expert Budwig's official verdict was "trans fats were not suitable for human consumption," an opinion written in 1951, three years before I started slurping trans fat in my baby formula. For this dietary insight, along with all her other decidedly unpopular views, Frau Budwig was impugned, sued, ridiculed, and consigned to the ash heap of fringe scientific extremism.

This doesn't mean she was wrong, just that she was wrong for her time, and she was way ahead of her time in building in a delivery system for fatty acids. In describing this, Frau Budwig likened the unsaturated hydrogen bonds in fatty acids to frayed sections on a length of thread. If you draw that thread through water the frayed sections more readily absorb liquid, or dye in that liquid, and in the same way electron-rich double carbon bonds in an unsaturated fatty acid pull at electron-hungry polar molecules in the surrounding solution of proteins and water.

This relatively weak but notable attraction is the force behind lipoproteins, which form when very long and twisted proteins link to and shroud fatty acids in a water soluble sheath. The protein-covered fat now dissolves in water, and lipoproteins are your body's main delivery system for carrying fat in blood. By providing the proper proteins along with highly unsaturated fatty acids conditions are conducive to creating quickly digested lipoproteins, which dissolve directly into the bloodstream and follow chemical messages for delivery to the cells that need them most.

A gel cap of shelf-stored fish or flax oil just isn't the same.

First off, the longer highly unsaturated fatty acids have been stored at room temperature, the less likely it is that the high energy bonds survive. Second off, I've tried eating gel caps of fish oil. It was awful. I'd pop a couple caps in the morning, the next day I'd still be burping like a Norwegian herring fisherman, which is not conducive to second dates.

It's about what you eat, and it's about how much you eat, but it's also about how much you digest. You can eat all the vitamin capsules in the world but if your piss is bright yellow how much good have you really done? So, now, since this is a science book, it's time for a chemistry experiment.

Take one cup red newts...

Just kidding.

Take one teaspoon of flax oil, or about a ninth of your daily allotment of oil in a fairly low fat diet, and then mix that teaspoon of flax oil with either two teaspoons of cottage cheese or four teaspoons of yogurt. Either way, the ratio of protein to fats is correct, and, since you're going to drink this science project, I recommend yogurt.

Dump the fat and oil in a blender, give it a whirl. The fat's gone. It's not like oil and plain water. The fat has dissolved into the protein. It's chemistry. It's like sending your cells supplies by FedEx instead of book rate; the materials get there much faster and require less handling.

Even so, flax oil and yogurt are a poor excuse for a tasty dish, and let's face it, we all love a tasty dish, at least in my house. So I add bananas, frozen strawberries that have been partially thawed in the microwave, orange juice, and a dash of soy milk, then churn it into a chilled smoothie, and call it breakfast. Unless I've been out carousing and playing music the night before, then I might have sausage and eggs.

It defies logic, but a greasy breakfast is the best cure for a hangover I ever found.

The point is that when it comes to diet, you have to be reasonable. You have to be you. I'll never have the discipline to count calories, not in a million years. Plus, if you want to live a semi-normal life, it's impossible to give up processed food completely.

Still, the vast bulk of what I now eat is fresh vegetables and fruit, whole grains and beans. I do make a diligent effort to avoid the empty calories of foods containing highly processed oils, and I cook with raw olive oil and butter because the fatty acids characteristic of these foods stand up well to the heat of cooking and provide a blend of nutrients. I used to eat meat once or twice a day, now I eat it three or four times a week, and when I do, I get the good stuff, like grass fed buffalo or wild caught salmon.

You see, you can be smart about diet, but you still have to live. Whatever you do to balance your diet is going to work better if you have some fun along the way. In this regard Frau Budwig again voiced strong opinions with comments like: "If a woman has a very poor marriage, and has to deal with suppression and taunts from her husband day in and day out, then I cannot help her with (cottage cheese)-flax oil."

I hear that.

The full-on Budwig anticancer protocol calls for the elimination of "respiratory poisons" such as insecticides and falling-out-of-love; it also places great emphasis on the healing power of sunshine. Contemporary research shows sunshine and the associated production of vitamin D do indeed affect many fundamental bodily processes, but Frau Budwig saw the effects of the sun on human health quite differently.

To her way of thinking, the human body is an antenna, and the electron-rich highly unsaturated fatty acids are the foods that provide the electrons that tune the antenna that draws in the power of sun, "thus causing a recharging of the living substance—especially of the brain and nerves."

It seems to me you pay a little more attention to your elders, especially if they've been nominated for Nobel Prizes. Plus, in convincing anecdotal evidence, Frau Budwig, taking her own advice, lived to be an ever feisty ninety-three years old. She railed to the end against what she called "electron thieves," and if these thieves thought electrons worth stealing, I determined to understand what it was they stole.

Electrons

The first thing to understand about electrons is that you can't understand them. Not completely. Not on the scale at which we live our lives. Electrons exist on the subatomic scale where nothing is absolute because everything is relative, and it is at the level of electrons that the force of life that is you is played out.

"I don't have any energy."

How many times have we heard that?

But what does it really mean?

And can you fix it with a five hour drink?

Just as our bodies are conglomerations of cells our energies are conglomerations of electrons, and electrons are just small enough and just fast enough to forever blur the distinction between particles of matter and waves of energy. If you shoot an electron through a single slit onto a screen it hits like a bullet, splat. But if you take a bunch of electrons, and shoot them through a partition containing two slits, the electrons show up as an interference wave pattern on the screen behind the slits.

In the first case, a single electron acts like a particle.

In the second case, a bunch of electrons together act like waves.

The original double slit experiment was performed with candles rather than electrons in the early eighteenth century, and caused an about face in the direction of physics because it showed light was a wave as opposed to the particle predicted by Sir Isaac Newton. Many follow-up experiments ensued, culminating in 1873 when the physicist James Maxwell synthesized separate data on electricity and magnetism into elegant equations showing visible light was part of a larger spectrum of electromagnetic waves that universal constants demanded would move at 186,000 miles per second.

Light remained a wave for about thirty years, at which point the then patent clerk Albert Einstein boomeranged the wave versus particle debate on the nature of light full circle. Einstein won a Nobel Prize for demonstrating that while light might be a wave, it was also composed of discrete energy packets he called *photons*. On the quantum scale energy is distributed like particles, but travels like waves. Electrons and photons aren't particles or waves, they're something in between.

I can understand that. It's weird, but it's not that weird.

Here's where it gets really weird.

Technology progressed over the next fifty or so years until it became possible to shoot electrons not in streams, but individually. Scientists found that if you take single electrons, and fire them one at a time through two slits, the electrons no longer impact on the screen like single bullets that went through one slit or the other slit. Instead, the individual electrons show up as an interference pattern of waves.

Electrons that went through the slits at different times, and therefore could not have interfered with each other, nonetheless create an interference pattern. Somehow, each electron is interfering with itself. The most plausible explanation, which isn't all that plausible, is that each electron went through both holes at once. This would be a handy trick to master because you could be in two places at once. You could be fishing and painting the house

The Double Slit Experiment

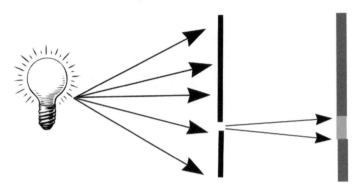

The original double slit experiment was performed to settle the dispute about whether light was a particle or a wave. Light passes through a single slit like a series of particles, and impacts on the screen behind the slit in a single band of brightness. When two slits are opened, however, rather than a single band of light behind each slit, an alternating series of dark and light bands appears across the entire screen, a pattern that is characteristic of wave interference. When the crests of two waves coincide the energy of the waves reinforce each other, and appear as a band of light. When the crest of one wave coincides with the trough of another wave the energy of the waves causes the waves to cancel each other out, and appears as a band of darkness, a phenomenon that is only possilbe if light acts as a wave as well as a particle.

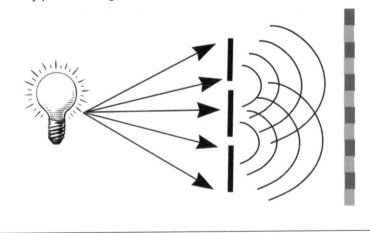

at the same time, but only as long as nobody knew where you were, because at the level of electrons if it's certain you're in one place then you can no longer be in the other.

If you equip the double slit experiment with measuring devices so that you can determine through which of the two slits the electron passed on its way to the screen, then the electron no longer goes through both holes. If you pin down the location of each electron as it passes through the double slit partition the interference pattern disappears, and the electrons once again impact like bullets in a single strip of energy on the screen behind each slit.

This led a physicist named Richard Feynman, who is generally the smartest guy in the room no matter who else is in the room, to conclude that when electrons travel from point A to point B they do it by taking every conceivable path. They go straight from A to B, but they also go by way of the grocery store, the constellation Aquarius, and all other possible paths. This would be some trick all by itself, but the kicker is that electrons take all these paths in the same instant of time. According to Feynman, electrons are everywhere at once.

This is even better than magic. Electrons can do things Harry Potter can't, and electrons exist only because they are more likely to be found in some places rather than all the other places. No matter where you go there you are, and wherever you are, you're there because the chances are high that you'll be there.

This is probability theory, and when it comes to atoms, according to another famous physicist named Max Planck, there is a high probability electrons will be found at certain distances from the atomic nucleus at particular energy states called *orbits*. Electrons assume orbits because the distance around the sphere allows them to circle the nucleus in a whole number of their particular wavelengths. Every time an electron jumps from one orbit to another in

Single Electrons and the Double Slit

Single electrons fired through a single slit impact on the screen like particles in a single band of energy.

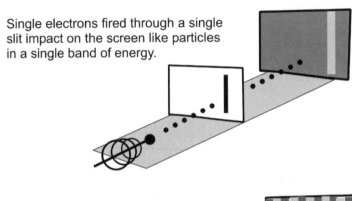

Electrons fired one at a time through two slits produce bands characteristic of wave interference.

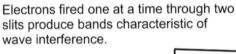
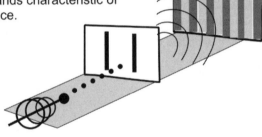

Single electrons, when you measure to see which slit they passed through, no longer create wave intereference patterns.

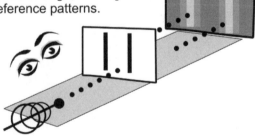

your body—which is all the time as your cells process chemicals—energy is transferred in the form of an electromagnetic wave.

This is the energy of life.

When a cell burns glucose in the presence of oxygen, electrons jump from high energy orbits to low energy orbits, thus releasing energy. When cells process raw materials into finished products, electrons (overall) jump from low energy orbits to high energy orbits, thus requiring energy. This is the force that ultimately drives you, and if it's in balance, so are you.

The electromagnetic radiation that permeates your cells is a variation on the same theme as the electromagnetic radiation that comes from the sun. Either way, the energy travels in waves much like the waves that travel through water in a lake. A wave in a lake passes energy from molecule to molecule. Individual water molecules don't move from point to point, instead energy is transferred as the water molecules rise and fall in the motion of the wave as the energy crosses the lake.

In the same way electromagnetic waves pass through the vacuum of space on perpendicular fields of electricity and magnetism according to the equations put forth by James Maxwell. The individual electromagnetic fields don't move from point to point, the standing fields instead simply fluctuate in intensity as they pass along the energy of the wave. This is possible because moving electric fields create corresponding magnetic fields, while moving magnetic fields create corresponding electric fields.

A power generator makes use of falling water or coal-derived steam to spin coils of conductive wire within a magnetic field, thus producing electricity. Audio tape stores information in strips of magnetism of varying directions and intensities; this magnetism, when passed over coils of wire, induces electrical current that can be reproduced as the sound of music. Electricity begets magnetism, magnetism begets electricity, and electromagnetic waves, as they travel through time, essentially create their own self-propagating, three-dimensional grid of electricity and magnetism out of the fabric of space as they pass.

In human terms, it would be as if you were on a road trip in your new car, hurtling along the electromagnetic highways, and at every increment of the journey you make a new car and abandon the last one. Your energy travels, but the cars don't, and these waves ride the electromagnetic grid in a continuum that for scientific convenience is artificially described by the length between the crests of the waves.

The electromagnetic waves with the longest wavelengths and lowest energies are called *radio waves,* with distances between crests that begin at about the size of a baseball and extend theoretically to the length of the universe. High energy gamma rays are at the opposite end of the electromagnetic spectrum, with distances between wave crests beginning at a trillionth of a meter, on the order of the size of atomic nuclei, and wavelengths that decrease from there.

In between, in order of increasing wavelengths, lie the energies known as microwaves, infrared radiation, ultraviolet radiation, and x-rays. Between infrared and ultraviolet radiation, at wavelengths on the order of the size of a large virus or small bacteria, lies the most familiar form of electromagnetic radiation, visible light. All electromagnetic radiation travels at the same speed, the speed of light, or 186,000 miles per second, which is also the cosmic speed limit in the universe as we know it.

Electromagnetic radiation never speeds up and it never slows down as it creates its own transmission matrix at the speed of light. Light always travels at the speed of light, and the question the sixteen-year-old patent clerk Albert Einstein asked was what would happen if you chased after a beam of light.

Could you catch it?

According to Newton, you can catch up with a beam of light. According to Maxwell, you can't. According to Einstein, no matter how fast or slow your motion at a constant velocity, electromagnetic waves will always catch up with you at the speed of light. If you're standing still, and a spaceship is moving at a million miles an hour, and a bomb goes off half way between you and the spaceship, then both you and the people in the spaceship will see the light at the same time. No matter how fast you go, the speed of light is always the same, and if the speed of light doesn't change then something else must, and it turns out that what changes is time and space.

If you go fast enough, clocks slow down while rulers grow shorter. This is the world in which electrons live, and cellular life is defined by a constant flow of electrons and an accompanying flood of electromagnetic radiation. This energy is intrinsic to life itself, and, to me, the question isn't whether this pervasive bath of incessantly fluctuating electromagnetism affects our cells, as how could it not?

Still, it's one thing to believe in a relative universe based in uncertainty, where nothing is absolute because probability reigns. It's one thing to concede against logic that electrons just might be everywhere at once, and it's a whole other thing to stand up in a room full of people and attempt to manifest the energy of those electrons in a healthful fashion by pretending you're a reptile.

Qigong

Q*i*, pronounced chee, in Chinese medical philosophy, is a ubiquitous force that permeates the universe, moves the planets, and condenses into matter, including you and me. *Gong*, pronounced gong, refers generally to the process of bettering yourself by working at something. *Qigong*, or chee-gong, is the idea that you can consciously draw energy from the universe and store it as a life force by imitating the movements of certain animals, including the turtle.

"A turtle?" I said.

It's not what you think of when you think of a power animal.

"I was kind of hoping for an eagle," I said. "Or a bear."

I was doing what I do when I'm uncomfortable, making a joke. The teacher of the qigong class in which I had enrolled, whom we'll call Ms. Qi because it's a name that blends east and west, was having none of it.

"For you," she said, "…perhaps a mosquito."

All right. I can take a hint.

People who like sawing fiddles, picking guitars, and claw-hammering banjos come from every social and economic stratum. I'd never much advocated Chinese medicine but I had long-time musical friends, including Ms. Qi, who did, and at their collective insistence I'd joined a class in qigong. What the heck, I figured, I had nothing to lose. Plus, lots of people swear by acupuncture. On the other hand, I'd been raised to be midwestern leery of quack-pot Chinese medicine, and this definitely qualified.

"Be the turtle," continued Ms. Qi, "by assuming the characteristics the turtle embodies. Slow, round, smooth, durable; envision these features in yourself..."

A dozen or so of us were learning Turtle Longevity Qigong, a discipline that explores the premise that since turtles live very long lives, people can too. The underlying principle is that we can learn from the world around us, and the first six-part form in this particular flavor of qigong is called Watching the Turtle.

This form—or series of exercises—reputedly works on the surface layers of the body. It is meant to cleanse energy meridians and open acupuncture points, thus making it easier for energy to flow, and it begins when you close your eyes.

The first time it's hard not to roll your eyes instead.

Now, standing, arms limp at your sides, touch the tip of your tongue to the roof of your mouth to complete a vital energy orbit between body and brain. Next relax limb by limb, and visualize a golden turtle about the size of a basin on the ground three feet in front of you. In your mind's eye, you and the turtle are at the seashore. Waves are splashing, hypnotically, and the golden turtle qi flows into you until...

You become the turtle.

Good...

Now you're ready to begin.

"Turtle Spinning Freely on Top of the Water..."

This is the action you now imagine and imitate, and our class followed Ms. Qi's lead like a bunch of baby turtles. One arm goes forward while the other goes back, like you're walking, except now you're swimming. Think flippers here, slide out, push back, your hands carving circles instead of lines. Arm swings to the rear finish with a slight hand punch to the bottom of the spine, arm swings to the front finish with a slight hand punch to the abdomen somewhat north of the gonads.

Each light double punch is meant to loosen the flow of energy through the lower *dan tian* (don tee-en), an energy storage vessel that resides in your lower trunk. For inscrutable reasons turtle exercises are repeated in multiples of 33, but by the time we got to 99 arm swings I'd worked up a bit of a sweat, so maybe that's the point.

After a moment to relax, the form continues into the next exercise:

"Turtle Swimming in Deep Water..."

Here, I had what can only be described as a flashback. I was probably nine or ten years old and skin diving with my family on the coral reefs off the Florida coast. I'd just put on my face mask and when a green turtle half as big as me popped up next to our rented boat, I jumped first and thought second.

"Whoa," I thought.

I had a good hold on him and it seemed inconceivable those tiny flippers could move that huge shell so fast that the rushing current tore the mask from my face. Since then I'd seen plenty of turtles swimming in deep water. I knew them well...

"Ninety-seven, ninety-eight, ninety-nine."

Whoa.

Where was I?

"Golden Turtle Splashed by Waves..."

Three steps forward, three steps back, a helpless turtle washing in the surf, don't try and control the waves, instead let the waves control you.

"Ninety-seven, ninety-eight, ninety-nine..."

There's something to be said for repetitive motion. It's soothing, like swimming, and if nothing else it's exercise. I never knew turtles worked so hard until I tried being one, but Chinese medicine is all about balance, and, in the next part of the form, all you exercise is your mind.

"Golden Turtle Resting in a Cave..."

Now you meditate while visualizing your lower dan tian as a golden turtle in a golden cave. The golden turtle pulls in energy from the universe around you, and as the energy accumulates, it is stored in the golden cave for future use.

At least that's the theory.

The technique involves emptying your mind of extraneous thoughts but in tasks involving meditation my mind is regrettably resilient to emptying. I was supposed to be feeding the golden turtle; instead I was sneaking looks at the women in the mirror.

It was better than thinking about the medical bills I couldn't pay.

As for the mirror, it was eight feet high, thirty feet long, and a remnant of this classroom's previous incarnation as a dance studio. It covered a whole wall, and for the past hour had featured the reflection of fine-looking women in tights and clingy tops bending, bouncing, swinging, and swaying. It was the kind of voyeurism I'd always found at least enjoyable and usually inspiring, but at this point I'd been deprived of testosterone for about two months, and rather than lust I found...

I knew I was lying when I tried to tell myself I cared...

And, wondering what it was that I had become, I would remember:

"Oh, right, the golden turtle..."

In the practice of qigong the top of the head, the soles of the feet, and the palms of the hands are akin to transfer points where outside energy is most readily absorbed into the body. I'd try to imagine it, to see and feel the energy from my hands, head, and feet converging on the cave in my belly, my turtle glowing so golden bright you could see it from space, all lit up like the Las Vegas strip.

And then I'd think about that last time in Vegas…

You can see the problem I have with meditation.

In this simplest form of the turtle qigong, following meditation, you then place your hands over the cave in your belly. This allows your hands to absorb some of the energy you have just stored, and the action is apparently sexually specific, maybe a right brain / left brain kind of a thing; at any rate Ms. Qi instructed the men to put their right hand over their left, while women were to put their left hand over the right.

Without testosterone, which hand went where?

It can all get so confusing.

"That heat in your hands is the qi…now wipe it on your face."

The final part of this form involves a self-administered massage of your scalp and face, paying particular attention to acupoints in your eyes and ears. The massage ends when you place both hands back on your lower dan tian, take a deep breath, and then raise your hands to rub open your eyes.

After you blink a couple of times you're probably going to smile.

Because you feel better.

At least I did.

Five years later I still do the turtle a few to several times a week, but furtively, because, even though I'm supposed to be dead, I still worry about what the neighbors might think. It could be nothing more than the meditation and exercise that makes me feel better, but for several reasons I've come to believe it's more than that.

As one example, the energy access point in the arch of the foot is an acupressure point called *yong quan*, or bubbling spring, and at times following a turtle session my springs are hot pots. Something is going on, something I can feel, a distinct and localized burning sensation in an area about the size of a pencil eraser that lasts a few to several minutes.

Is that qi?

And what the heck is qi anyway?

External Qi

Practitioners of traditional Chinese medicine believe we all have "internal qi," and that a proper flow of this energetic life force is essential to good health. Some gifted practitioners of qigong, following years of dedicated practice, are said to be able to consciously focus and project this vital energy so as to affect the world around them, a phenomenon described as "external qi."

May the force be with you.

It's a claim right out of the training manual for Jedi knights.

"Prove it!" decried a host of medical authorities.

Proof was hard to come by in China during the 1960s and 1970s because Chairman Mao, in furthering the Cultural Revolution, saw knowledge as a threat to his power. Mao persecuted wisdom of all types, and during the ensuing reign of terror anyone from university professors to practitioners of qigong faced exile or death. Edicts were enforced by idealist youths enrolled in the Red Army, and enacted by the Gang of Four, an advisory group that included Mao's concubine, which just goes to show it's good work if you can get it.

Mao's death in 1976 ended the social devastation of the Cultural Revolution, and formal investigation of qi as an energy force began in 1978 at the Shanghai Institute of the Atomic Nucleus, and continued through 1979 at the Shanghai Academy of Chinese Medicine. In all, over nine hundred experiments were performed, and these sessions typically began with a qi master who would first meditate to store energy.

The acupoint toward the bottom of your palm called *laogong* is an entry point for energy during the practice of qigong. In an expert's hand it is also an exit point, and these experiments typically continued as the qi master, now full of stored energy, extended his palm, and usually sweating profusely with the effort involved, shot qi through the laogong like Spiderman shoots his web at objects like radiation sensitive screens.

These screens included the element germanium, which, by virtue of its particular arrangement of electrons, is the metal of choice to detect far infrared radiation with wavelengths of 50-240 microns. Qi masters, aiming their palms (or sometimes fingers) from distances of 0.5 meters to 2 meters, were consistently able to activate the germanium target in repeatable fashion.

As you might imagine, this caused quite a stir.

Follow-up experiments showed the laogong had a positive electric charge when emitting qi, and a negative charge at rest. Measurements at the *neiguan*, an acupoint on the inside of the arm just above the wrist, showed electrical resistance was "drastically reduced" during the emission of qi, supporting practitioner's claims that they can "feel" the qi flowing down their arms and out their palms as they emit energy.

In other experiments qi masters modulated both frequency (distance between waves) and intensity (height of wave) of microwave radiation from up to five meters away. Another practitioner aiming at a voltmeter placed 50 centimeters from his palm generated an electric current of 27.5 millivolts, about the energy required to run brain cells or electromagnetic switches in devices such as thermostats. Collaboration between the Chinese Geologic

University, the Beijing Medical University, and the Institute of Earth Physics associated qi with detectable magnetic properties. Experiments at the Chinese Institute of Space Medical Engineering found qigong healer groups emitted infrasound at frequencies lower than 16 Hz.

Experiments like these were designed to describe exactly what kind of energy qi was, but qi turned out to be as difficult to pin down as electrons. Qi wasn't just one thing, it was many things, or, if you believe the philosophy, it's everything.

Or, if you don't believe the philosophy, it's nothing.

What I find hard to disbelieve is the sheer bulk of accumulated evidence on the existence of external qi. There are too many reports on too many effects by too many respected scientists at too many prestigious research centers for it to be collusion, yet these studies have been largely ignored by western medicine for three main reasons.

First, some studies were well conceived and administered, while others were scientifically suspect, and the good work has been denounced along with the poor.

Second, well designed experiments generally measure the effects of changes in one parameter at a time. Change enzyme X, and the rate of reaction Z increases. Change enzyme X and temperature T, and you can't know whether it was X or T that changed reaction Z. Conclusive studies reduce equations to the level of one cause and one effect, and whatever qi is, it's more than that.

Third, results aren't scientifically valid until they are repeated in independent conditions, and any activity involving consciousness will never be exactly reproducible every time, because consciousness constantly changes, as any golfer can relate.

Suppose you just hit your drive 250 yards straight down the fairway. (Nice one.) You did it once, you should be able to do it again. The ability is within you, but no matter how good you are, you can't do it every time. Even the best professional golfers can't hit the fairway all the time, and it's harder under pressure.

Qi practitioners exhibit similar singularity. Baseline ability varies radically from one practitioner to the next, within the same person from day to day, and even from one moment to the next. Many experiments show that the amount of measurable energy exuded tends to decrease as practitioners tire over the course of individual trials, and then increases again after they rest and have something to eat.

My guess is their cuisine didn't include Twinkies.

There is general agreement among qi masters that, particularly when first requested to do so, they have difficulty focusing energy on inanimate objects such as germanium sensors. They describe qi as a life force more easily directed at life, and over the years experiments on the effects of external qi have been performed on a variety of animals, including rodents, flies, rabbits, fish, dogs, toads, and pigs.

One such 1997 study began with eighteen young pigs. The pigs weighed in at about twenty to thirty pounds when their spinal cords were cut to induce the "standard model of spinal paralysis," and three randomly-selected groups of six pigs each were then exposed to varying amounts of external qi.

The first group received a first treatment twelve hours after spinal injury, three times a day for the first week, then twice a day for the next eighty-four days. The second group did not begin treatment until seven days after the initial injury, but then received treatment twice a day for the next eighty-four days. The third group served as a control and received no treatment at all, and at the end of the ninety day period not one of the qi deprived pigs in the control group could so much as stand up.

In the second group, by contrast, five of six pigs could stand, and one could run. The pigs in the first group that received early and more overall treatment fared best: all six pigs could walk, and two of them could run and jump. It seems pigs, like people, are not created equal. It is likely qi affects different individuals to different degrees, but the overlying results of this experiment remain compelling.

All pigs in the first group could walk; no control pigs could stand.

Again, these are the kind of results that get your attention.

Nerve repair that cures paralysis is generally considered infeasible by western medicine, and when I read that study I thought of my friend Doug. Doug was once the National Football League defensive player of the year, an Adonis of a man who broke his neck skiing and ended up a paraplegic. I just saw Doug last month, a vibrant spirit struggling to push his wheelchair through the grass, and I had to wonder what might have happened if he'd received external qi early and often.

Maybe nothing, but...

Did dancing around like a turtle do me any real good?

Could it help cure my cancer?

Dozens of studies at dozens of hospitals have shown the application of external qi deters the growth of lung, liver, breast, blood, spleen, and gastric cancer cells. Over fifty of these reports were summarized in a 2002 paper out of the Robert Wood Johnson Medical School in New Jersey. Studies were selected according to "stringent criteria," including systematic data collection and control group comparison, and include *in vitro* studies on cultured cells, *in vivo* studies on tumors in mice, and human studies.

For instance, in one study cultured laboratory cervical cancer cells were exposed to twenty minutes of external qi; the treated cells showed an average 31 percent reduction in growth compared to untreated control cells. Other experiments on other cultured cancer cell lines showed reductions in growth of 25-60 percent in response to various applications of external qi; in an example of a slightly more complex in vitro experiment, 96 samples of cultured human cancer cells were broken into four groups.

One group received no treatment, one group received conventional gamma ray radiation therapy, one group received external qi, and the final group received both external qi and conventional radiation therapy. Cancer cells receiving either external qi or conventional radiotherapy showed similar reductions in the initial growth rates, while combining qi with conventional radiotherapy suppressed cell growth by an additional 58 percent over either treatment alone.

Many in vivo experiments show external qi has an effect on cancer implanted in mice. In one typical study 114 nude mice were injected with human cancer. Mice receiving ten to thirty minutes of external qi a day, after twenty days, had average tumor volumes of 2.2 cubic centimeters as opposed to 6.3 for control.

That's well over half the cancer that never got growing.

After a while, you have to think there might be something to this qi stuff.

Dozens of similar experiments at institutions ranging from the Chinese Navy General Hospital to the Chinese Institute of Biology have shown similar reductions in tumor mass, volume, and metastasis. For instance, in a study at the Zhongshan Medical University cultured liver cancer was transplanted into thirty mice, which were then randomly separated into three groups of ten. One group of mice received ten minutes of treatment from a qi master at a distance of four to six inches every other day for a total of forty minutes in four sessions, one group received sham treatment by a qi faker imitating the actions of the qi master, and the last group of mice received no treatment.

The tumors were removed and weighed in a blind fashion at day ten or eleven following initial implantation. Over three separate trials, tumor growth in the qi-treated group was inhibited an average of about 75 percent as compared to control and sham-treated groups; researchers estimated there was a one-in-ten-thousand probability these results could be due to chance. Microscopic examination of the qi-treated cancer cells revealed many features that would lead to lower tumor growth, including nuclear fragmentation, swollen mitochondria, and the remains of cells destroyed by apoptosis.

Of course, it's one thing to be a master of qi.

It's another to be me.

Or thee.

Qi masters, in describing their skills, speak of strengthening *yi* (yee, or conscious intent) through meditation to create an "empty mind without desire." This allows release from the "socialized self," the source of all stress, and return to the "original self," a state in which they are open vessels for the absorption and transfer of energy.

Is this something regular people can do?

Or is it just a bunch of mumbo-jumbo?

Again, studies indicate regular people who practice qigong can help themselves, both with higher survival rates and lower rates of side effects. For instance, at the Henan Medical University 186 post-surgical cancer patients were divided into four random groups. A control group received no further treatment following surgery; a second group received conventional chemotherapy; a third group received treatment with Chinese herbs; and a fourth group received Chinese herbs plus a daily dose of qigong.

One-year survival rates were similar for all groups, but five years later the survival rates were 21 percent for surgery alone, 25 percent for surgery plus chemotherapy, 26 percent for surgery plus Chinese herbs, and 36 percent for the group that received both Chinese herbs and qigong treatment. The median survival rate for the qi plus herb group was 48 months, as compared to 30 months for the control group.

It is important to emphasize that the patients in this study (and most studies on the effects of external qi) had highly advanced cancers. When the noose is around your neck an additional eighteen months is an eternity, perhaps long enough to meet your new grandchild. It is a time when quality of life is important, and this study found generally negligible side effects associated with the Chinese herb and qi treatment, while the side effects associated with chemotherapy are all too well documented.

Another study examined the relative effects of qigong and chemotherapy on quality of life by separating 123 patients with advanced stage III and IV cancers into two groups. One group received traditional chemotherapy, the other received chemotherapy plus two hours of qigong a day for three months. At the end of the treatment period 82 percent of the qi group regained strength, 63 percent improved appetite, and 33 percent were diarrhea free, as compared to 10 percent, 10 percent, and 6 percent of the group that did not practice qigong.

This same study found that an indicator of immune function improved 14 percent in the qi group, while it decreased 8 percent in the non-qi group. Several other studies show qi treatment increases immune function, including levels of associated proteins and actual counts of immune cells. Many other studies at many other hospitals found patients who practiced qigong had improved rates of DNA repair, increased white and red blood cell counts, and improved blood flow, particularly through the capillaries, which are crucial to the transfer of oxygen and energy to individual cells.

There's that oxygen again.

The multifaceted nature of qi is further indicated in an experiment performed at the Tongji Medical University. In this study three qi masters were asked to direct their will at test tubes with the intent of changing the rate of a chemical reaction, the oxidation of glucose. Five hundred trials later the masters had increased the rate of the reaction an average of 400 percent, while the standard deviation on control group reactions was less than 5 percent. The effects were detectable at a distance of 2 to 10 meters, stronger when closer, undetectable at 12 meters, and effective whether or not the qi master was facing the equipment.

That external qi apparently affects respiration in live cells as well as chemical reactions in test tubes was demonstrated at the National Yang Ming Medical College, in one of several studies that seem to validate practitioner's claims that the application of qi has both positive and negative effects.

In this study a qi master emitted either "peaceful mind qi" or "destroying mind qi" at cultured sperm cells. In each case qi was emitted from the laogong at distances of 10, 20, 30, 40, and 50 centimeters. The effect was greatest at a distance of 20 centimeters, where ten minutes of "peaceful mind qi" increased rates of respiration by 28 percent and DNA synthesis by 12 percent. The changes were more pronounced for a mere two minutes of "destroying mind qi," which decreased cellular respiration rates by 53 percent and DNA synthesis by 22 percent (all numbers relative to control.)

Another experiment, performed at the Center for Immunological Research in Beijing and published in the *Chinese Nature Journal,* was also designed to determine what effect, if any, the intent of the practitioner would have on the growth of bacteria.

The experiment was so simple the data is hard to dispute. A qi master, palm out, extruded qi from his laogong at Petri dishes full of cultured E. coli bacteria. Relative to control dishes that received no treatment, bacterial growth was inhibited 45-91 percent in response to "negative" external qi, and bacterial growth was accelerated 2.3 to 6.9 times when basking in the glow of "positive" external qi.

These results are the range of an experiment over twenty trials, and the numbers are huge, even at the low end. At the high end, 6.9 times is 690 percent, and a 90 percent swing in one direction and a 690 percent swing in the other direction is the difference between a tumor that weighs 0.1 ounce or 6.9 ounces, which places the potential difference between the power of positive and negative thought on the scale of orders of magnitude.

It's easy to impugn these numbers. They're too good to be true. The idea that you can use your mind to direct the flow of energy in your body in a positive or a negative manner is a tough pill to swallow if you've grown up on a steady diet of western rationalism. On the other hand, some studies examining patients who practiced qigong reported cases of "complete remission from late-stage or metastasized cancer, which is considered an impossible result through the use of conventional medicine alone."

To me, the nature of qi is no less improbable than the nature of electrons. In the double slit experiment, if matter is seen in Eastern terms as condensed qi, it is possible to visualize the electron "evaporating" into both slits at once. Maybe qi is like water, and it can exist as the energetic equivalent of either liquid or vapor, and each phase has specific properties. A cloud couldn't be more different than an ocean, but it's still water, and when it comes to the universe, it's all qi.

The laws of physics demand our collective cells create collective electromagnetic energies yet, even in China, let alone the rest of the world, most doctors disregard the notion that consciousness controls a subtle human energy. One such skeptic was David Eisenberg from the Harvard Medical School, one of the first western doctors to visit China following the Cultural Revolution. He wrote a book about his experience, and it is convincing that something called qi might exist, simply because he went into the experience so unconvinced.

At the time, so close to the death of Mao, the qigong masters were still mostly underground. They had been persecuted for years, and Doctor Eisenberg's initial encounters were clandestine affairs in back alleys and basements, like something out of spy books. Nonetheless, Doctor Eisenberg describes many experiences in his travels, including clairvoyance, that "seemed to suggest the existence of qi," but what he (like most of us) craved was the ultimate parlor trick.

Doctor Eisenberg wanted to see a human being move an object using nothing more than their mind. After repeated requests over several months the Chinese administration at the time finally sanctioned a meeting at a government laboratory with a man named Comrade Lin, who, in a closed room, attempted to direct his energy at a dart comprised of three feathers suspended from a string.

With his palm about three feet away from the dart, wearing a hospital mask so he couldn't move the dart with his breath, the veins in his neck and arms bulging, muscles trembling, sweating profusely, Comrade Lin rotated his palm clockwise. The dart did likewise. As the qi master rotated his palm the dart followed his motions; when he used both hands together the motions of the dart increased, and when he moved his hands back and forth the dart began to sway to and fro. Doctor Eisenberg describes how Comrade Lin then stepped back, visibly fatigued, ripped the mask from his face, and after decades of concealing his skill yelled:

"What do you think now?"

Too Many Ohms
in the Meridian

Human blood flows through a system of capillaries, arteries, and veins that permeate and connect all the hundred trillion cells in a typical body, and practitioners of Chinese medicine contend that human qi flows through a similar network of meridians. It is these meridians that the process of acupuncture reputedly stimulates and, for what it is worth, there is a vast amount of anecdotal evidence that acupuncture is effective.

For instance, I used to play in a country band, and Paul, our upright bass player, couldn't even hold his bass much less play it because of a pinched nerve in his neck. He tried pills, physical therapy, a chiropractor. Nothing helped. He was walking around with his ear nearly touching his shoulder before desperation finally conquered a deeply held aversion to all things Oriental, and he finally tried acupuncture.

I can still hear the surprise in Paul's voice.

"It worked," he said.

One of the great criticisms by western medicine of acupuncture is that the physical structures that could host the meridians have never been found. The needles go in, but into what? There's nothing there, not nerves anyway, and the aforementioned Doctor

David Eisenberg viewed claims that acupuncture was as effective as traditional anesthesia during a variety of surgical procedures skeptically.

He was therefore invited to watch an operation on a fifty-eight-year-old history professor, Comrade Lu, who had a chestnut-sized tumor of the pituitary. Such tumors so deep in the brain are generally removed through the nose, but this tumor was too big. To gain access the surgeons had to cut a four-inch-by-six-inch hole in the skull, and for anesthesia, they used acupuncture.

Doctor Eisenberg watched as a total of six needles were inserted into Comrade Lu: one in each eyebrow, two more in the left temple, and the final two needles went in the left shin and ankle. After each insertion the acupuncturist would ask:

"Do you have the qi?"

"Yes," or "No," answered the history professor.

If the answer was no, the needle was reinserted or twisted until Comrade Lu "felt" a physical sensation associated with the acupuncture point. These six needles, once qi was achieved, were then attached to wires that ended at a hand-painted black box containing a twelve-volt car battery and a transformer. Twenty minutes later, when the history professor was judged to be sufficiently sedated, the doctors sliced back three sides of a four-inch-by-six-inch flap of skin, and folded the tissue out of the way.

Holes were then drilled at the corners of the bare rectangle of exposed skull, and a wire bone saw was threaded between adjacent holes and pulled back and forth until a side was cut. Four sides later the brain was exposed, at which time the surgeons went at Comrade Lu's brain with scalpels. This whole time, in a procedure that lasted four hours, the history professor appeared alert and conscious, his head immobilized in a frame of steel tubes, and the surgeons encouraged Doctor Eisenberg to carry on a conversation (which I paraphrase) with the patient.

Doctor Eisenberg: "What's on your mind?"

Comrade Lu got the joke and laughed.

"I was just wondering what they would think of this procedure in a typical American hospital," he said.

Doctor Eisenberg was wondering the same thing and asked:

"Do you feel any pain? Anything at all?"

Comrade Lu: "No."

The brain itself doesn't have nerves that feel pain, but the skull, blood vessels, and skin do. That Comrade Lu could carry on a conversation while his brain was exposed certainly speaks toward the efficacy of acupuncture and the existence of the associated meridians, as do many contemporary studies.

The underlying premise of acupuncture is that a needle placed in one part of the body affects the flow of energy, resulting in changes to another part of the body. Body temperature—in both eastern and western medicine—is an important indicator of health, and in one contemporary study a high quality sensor was used to measure skin temperature changes in response to acupuncture.

A point on the lower inside leg, which would be expected to affect the stomach, was needled. Changes in skin temperature in the stomach region changed 0.5° -2.0° centigrade, while changes in skin temperature in the control region of the lower back, where no needles were inserted, were about 0.1° centigrade. These same researchers, in another paper, reported skilled practitioners were able to generate electrical currents in the meridians of up to about 100 millivolts.

After a while, no matter how western your roots, it's difficult to categorically dismiss the concept of energy meridians, which leaves the problem of what they are since nobody has ever found one. The simplest solutions are generally the best, and one intriguing hypothesis proposes that these meridians are composed of a first-rate conductor of electricity that all life possesses in abundance: water.

Maybe meridians were right there all along. Because of its polar nature, water has to conduct electricity. It can't do anything else. That's why you don't use a hair dryer while you're taking a shower. According to this theory, under the influence of electricity the meridians are composed of stable water clusters that line up (since electrical opposites attract) positive to negative and negative to positive.

In other words, your energy, as it flows, creates its own transmission medium out of charged water particles. In this, consider electromagnetic radiation, which creates its own transmission medium out of magnetism and electricity as it flows. Either way, the energy and the grid through which it flows are detectable only when a wave of energy is actually passing.

That's not so farfetched.

You can't find meridians when you cut open a cadaver, because qi is a life force, not a dead force. The flow is in your water, and water came first. Water is fundamental to the nature of cellular life on Earth and it is entirely plausible that qi, sometimes described as original energy, would flow in the original source material.

Water has a nature all its own, and in the ever changing yet inexorable way of flowing water it is easy to visualize meridians of energy trickling between cells. Tiny rivulets of energy join into creeks as they flow through tissue; creeks combine into rivers of flow between organs. The flow is sometimes buried deep within the body, at other locations the energy is so close to the surface it can be adjusted with the point of a needle or the pressure of a massage.

The only constant in that flow is change, from here to there and moment to moment, sometimes wide and shallow, sometimes narrow and deep. The current can be turbulent with back eddies, or it can be placid and continuous. Organisms and obstacles can be encountered along the way. A river can flood; a river can evaporate away to nothing, and, according to traditional Chinese medicine, so can your qi.

Yin, Yang, and You

So, maybe your back is against the wall. Western treatments haven't worked and you're willing to try anything. It may also be that the sum of the evidence has convinced you alternative treatments deserve a chance. Either way, this chapter is a primer on what you might encounter on a foray into the arena of traditional Chinese medicine.

According to this discipline your health is dependent on your qi, and there are three sources of qi. The first is the qi you are born with, your "prenatal" qi. Prenatal qi is stored in the kidneys, bestows individuality like DNA because everybody gets a different blend, and you're born with a lifetime's supply. Once your prenatal qi is gone you are too, and how you use that supply of qi is up to you.

You can think of prenatal qi as a bank account. You're born with some money in this bank, maybe a little, maybe a lot, depending on what your ancestors left you. You can blow your life's savings in a hurry, or you can stretch it out. No matter what, it takes some qi to live, but you don't have to constantly deplete the energy you're born with, because you can obtain supplemental life force along the way.

The second source of qi is the food you eat, and the third source is the air around you. In Chinese medicine, that's it. Eat good food, breathe good air, have good friends that fill that good air, and you're taking in qi. You can live off this supplemental energy, so you don't need to draw on the finite supply you were born with.

At a cellular level, this makes sense. Your cells eventually wear out like anything else, and can only reproduce so many times. Providing cells with the raw materials they need in the proportions they require means they won't have to work as hard to get their jobs done. Cells that don't work as hard are likely to last longer before they wear out, and if your cells last longer it follows that you might too.

Experts describe many subcategories of qi, but it always comes in two flavors, *yin* and *yang*. Yang qi is more male and daytime activity; while yin qi is more female and the quiet of night. In the same way that there can't be women without men, or light without dark, there can't be yin without yang, because they are two sides of the same coin, a coin as small as the universe, and as vast as you.

All yin, no matter how feminine, even Snow White, contains an element of yang. All yang, no matter how masculine, even Rambo, contains an element of yin. And that element of yin, no matter how minute, in turn contains an element of yang. Yin begets yang, and yang begets yin, on and on, ad infinitum.

In an oft-used analogy yang is the light side of a hill, while yin is the side of the hill in shadow. Yin and yang mutually create, control, and transform one another in the same way that, as the sun passes over the hill, light becomes shadow and shadow turns to light. The surface of the hill isn't perfectly smooth, so neither is the progression of shadow to light, and there are pockets within pockets within pockets.

Just as day and night have a yin and a yang, so does your body.

For instance, to a doctor of Chinese medicine, a problem in yin qi is associated with the gradual onset of chronic disease, which generally requires longer treatment with herbal therapy. Deficiencies in yang qi, on the other hand, are associated with the rapid onset of acute disease, and shorter term treatment with acupuncture.

A diagnosis will be based on the Eight Principles, which boil down to variations on only four: Interior and Exterior, Hot and Cold, Deficiency and Excess, and the ultimate in duality, yin and yang. That's simple enough, and a typical diagnosis in Chinese medicine begins with simple observation.

From your fingernails to your skin color to your posture, it all means something, and that there is art to this observation is revealed in the legend of a famous Chinese doctor with whom many students wished to study. Potential students who appeared at the doctor's door were seated in a room, and after a time presented with a dead fish and asked to write down their observations.

Left alone, some insulted students stalked off. Others observed for an hour or a day, and, in the absence of further instruction, left to study elsewhere. The students who eventually became apprentices stayed for weeks, studying the changing fish, noting details such as scale texture and eye film. These students were accepted because they were beginning to understand the unceasing change at the heart of the circle of life that is yin and yang, and because it is this attention to detail that makes a good doctor.

In practice, observation in a traditional medical appointment includes looking, listening, smelling, asking, and touching. A typical office visit might last an hour, and, as an example, suppose a patient arrives at a doctor's office:

"Please," says the doctor, "Sit down."

The patient coughs, the back of her hand to her mouth, then sighs.

"Thank you," she says. "The bus was so crowded..."

The doctor has already noted the patient's skin is pale not red, the cough shallow and weak as opposed to deep and full of phlegm. They chat, speaking of diet and social life because health is a matter of harmony in matters large and small; it is only later within the sphere of the overall picture that they arrive at specifics.

Doctor: "What seems to be your problem?"

Patient: "I can't sleep."

At this point in the west you are typically prescribed a sleeping pill, but, in eastern medicine, the goal isn't to make you sleep, it's to find out why you can't sleep. The goal is to root out the cause of this particular insomnia from the many possibilities that can impair sleep. Now suppose our hypothetical patient squeezes her slightly blue lips together as she suppresses a barely discernable belch. The faint lingering scent might not mean much to you or me, but, to the doctor, it is telling.

Doctor: "Do you have morning aches near the stomach?"

Patient: "Sometimes, yes, but more to the side."

The doctor then taps the abdomen here, there, a little higher, a little lower.

"Does it hurt more here....or here."

Patient: "Ah...higher...there...when it is bad...that is where it is worst."

Doctor: "And when you breathe deeply...is the pain worse?"

Specific, directed questions locate the imbalance in qi, interior or exterior, and the nature of the problem, hot, cold, damp or dry, yang or yin. Each question leads to the next, and at some point in the process, just like an old-fashioned visit to a western doctor, the eastern doctor is going to say something like:

"Please, now, may I see your tongue?"

To a trained observer the tongue can vary in color from white to yellow to red; it can be thick with mucous or dry with cracks, and conditions fluctuate from side to side and front to back. Some institutes of learning in traditional healing have models of hundreds of tongues, each tongue exhibiting characteristics that in turn are diagnostic of conditions in other parts of the body, all of which students are expected to learn.

For instance, a redder than normal tongue with a deep red tip and a yellow, greasy coating indicates an "excess of damp internal heat" in the lungs or heart, and symptoms such as pneumonia. In the case of our hypothetical patient, let's say her tongue is pale with a thin coating of mucous, the center dry and cracked. This indicates an overall deficiency in yang qi, and energy imbalances of the stomach or spleen.

Inflatable arm cuffs now have the job but I'm old enough to remember my pulse being taken by hand. This personal touch is fundamental to a diagnosis in traditional Chinese medicine, and a doctor uses three fingers to measure six pulses in each wrist, three pulses that are deep, and three pulses that are superficial.

Each of the twelve pulses (six in each wrist) correspond to a specific bodily organ or system, and the frequency, rhythm, strength, and volume of each pulse describe the relative status of qi in the associated systems. In the case of our patient who can't sleep, the superficial middle pulse in her right wrist is feeble, indicating a deficiency of energy in the stomach. The deep third pulse in the right wrist is barely detectable, indicating a deficiency in overall yang qi of the kidney. Overall, this leads the doctor to a diagnosis of weak "blood" or "body" qi—akin to anemia— and the reason the woman can't sleep is because her stomach has not been processing food well.

The doctor prescribes herbs and acupuncture that will treat this deficiency in the stomach, as opposed to herbs and acupuncture designed to help the woman sleep. This difference—the attempt to initially treat the root cause of the illness as opposed to the symptom—is a fundamental distinction between typical eastern and western approaches to medicine.

This really hit home with me.

Western medicine treats cancer like colds and insomnia, by targeting symptoms. We plug up runny noses; we prescribe powerful sedatives; we poison mutated cells. Depending on the severity of symptoms this may or may not make sense, but it makes no sense to believe this is where healing ends, and it makes even less sense to believe this is where healing begins.

I've read that in the old days there were Chinese doctors who were paid only if their patients stayed well. The emphasis was on preventative medicine, the idea that by the time you need a hospital it is already in many ways too late, and if we lived in such a world a foray into our health care system would be an entirely different affair.

Doctor: "I'm sorry those pills didn't work…you don't owe me a thing."

You: "Really?"

Doctor: "Would you pay a plumber if the faucet still leaks?"

When was the last time your health care experience went like that? Cost-cutting measures increasingly ensure you'll see a different doctor every day in a typical western hospital stay, while one skill at which every doctor and hospital I encountered along the way excelled was in the sending out of bills.

It's easy to see the benefits of treating the cause rather than the symptom of disease in a proactive cooperative effort between doctor and patient. It's less easy to see that cause and effect in terms of the Mutual Production Cycle of the Five Elements.

In traditional Chinese medicine, the Five Elements—Wood, Fire, Earth, Metal and Water—are born one from the other in the natural progression of the Mutual Production Cycle that continues until the end of time. Wood becomes fire, which leads to ashes in earth, which forges metal washed by the water that grows the wood. This is compared to spring growth maturing in summer heat that leads to earth's harvest and the cold metal of winter, which is washed away by spring rains that again bring growth.

The fundamental pattern of the five elements is shown in the accompanying diagram, and according to this theory, because it's all qi, each and every entity in the universe has a primary association with one or another of these elements. The element fire is linked to the color red, a scorched odor, a bitter taste, the sound of a laugh. Metal is associated with rice, a dry climate, grief, the direction west. Earth is associated with the color yellow, a fragrant smell, a sweet taste, and the sound of a song.

The sound of that song, you might be thinking, is Loony Tunes.

At first, I filed all this away with unicorns and dragons. It was ludicrous, yet as I came to believe that one of the mysterious ways in which electrons work is called qi, I began to see the five elements more as five energies. Get past the stereotypes of the physical substances and visualize the inherent differences in the underlying energies, and it is no great stretch to see how the crystalline nature of metal is very different from the inexorable flow of water, which is very different from the quick burning of fire.

The idea is that energy is everywhere in the universe. Everything we taste, smell, hear, touch, and see has a certain kind of energy of which we partake as we interact with the world around us. Change one thing and you change everything else. The goal is balance between yin, yang, and the five elements, and, in terms specific to health, each of these five energies is also thought to be associated with specific organs in your body.

The qi of wood is associated with the liver, fire with the heart, earth with the spleen, metal with the lungs, and water with the kidneys. The distinctive energies of each organ mutually produce and control each other as they flow through water-borne meridians, a process that is affected by another kind of qi, your mind.

The Five Elements of Energy

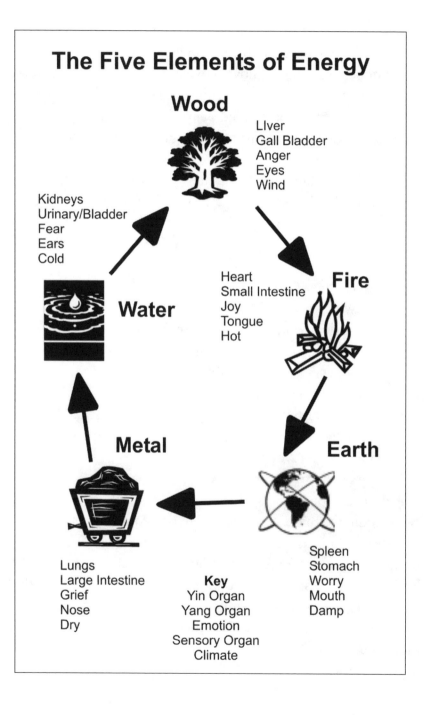

Wood

LIver
Gall Bladder
Anger
Eyes
Wind

Kidneys
Urinary/Bladder
Fear
Ears
Cold

Water

Heart
Small Intestine
Joy
Tongue
Hot

Fire

Metal

Earth

Lungs
Large Intestine
Grief
Nose
Dry

Key
Yin Organ
Yang Organ
Emotion
Sensory Organ
Climate

Spleen
Stomach
Worry
Mouth
Damp

There is no Cartesian separation of mind and body in Chinese medicine. It's all qi, part of the same whole. The conscious stimulation of healthful energy flow between organs becomes increasingly important in advanced forms of qigong, and by the end of my class, in a sitting form called Being the Turtle, a lot of what we did was simply meditate on the mutual production cycle as it related to our organs.

"Think of qi flowing...from the liver...to the heart...to the spleen...to the lungs... kidneys...wood...fire...earth...metal... water...liver...heart...spleen...lungs...kidneys..."

Ms. Qi's voice, always the same...slow...round...smooth...like a turtle:

"Any questions..."

"Yeah...what's a spleen?"

The organs in traditional Chinese medicine are composite structures of form and function that include associated meridians of associated energies. Again, it comes down to the idea that we function together, not apart, and outwardly different parts of the body share similarities because they share similar energies. In this, consider that an oak tree and a piano don't look anything alike, but they're both largely wood.

Of course, they're other things too.

And so are your organs, yin within yang within yin.

According to this theory, among myriad connections, the color and strength of the fingernails are said to be a window into the liver. The kidneys are related to both bones and baldness. The lungs include the sacks of alveoli we inflate every time we breathe, but also relate to skin and body hair. The heart pumps blood but is also linked to the tongue, while the spleen, the largest organ in the immune system, is energetically related to the mouth, lips, and digestion as a whole.

The five distinctive elemental energies are said to be in you and around you, constantly swapping out a yin and a yang as they flow, and it is this flow that governs your health. If the energies are in balance, you have a high resistance to the pathogens that constantly attack your body. Conversely, if the harmony is disrupted, then even weak pathogens can have virulent effects.

Energy imbalances can be caused by excesses such as wind, cold and wet; moods such as joy, anger, and anxiety; intemperance in eating and drinking; and too much or too little of sex, work, or exercise. As always, these pathogens tend to act upon one part of the body and manifest in another.

As an example, consider a person who is depressed: things are going poorly on the romantic front. This person can now be having both too much and too little sex at the same time: too much with him or herself and not enough with somebody else. It's a double imbalance with which your body is genetically ill equipped to cope, and while depression is a natural result, the solution probably isn't antidepressants.

Just because germs cause disease doesn't mean wind can't. Get two fat guys in your drift boat, try and row them well on a windy day; you too will know the power of the wind. Wind can suck the life right out of you. This is something every fishing guide knows. Wind is the worst, unless of course it's windy and rainy, which at the end of the day can lead to intemperance in drinking.

It's all connected. It's your world. You make the choices. In traditional Chinese medicine, you matter. Not only that, you *are* matter.

Which is simply condensed qi.

$E=mc^2$.

As I meditated on the turtle, consciously directing the flow of various energies between various organs, wood grew. It bent, it changed with humidity. I thought about how wood is hard to break but easy to cut, and how it burns. I thought about fire...how it heats my house, how it cycles forests to dirt...the earth as a crucible for the crystal lattice of the metals that tune in different frequencies of radiation...the water that makes life possible, the sound of a bubbling brook, and I thought about cancer.

I saw cancer cells drowning, burning. I hacked at them with a sharp metal blade, the dead mutants disappearing into the earth as I pissed them out. I filled my turtle with the longer infrared wavelengths of electromagnetism in the form of life-giving qi, and tried not to fret about the shorter wavelengths of electromagnetic radiation I was about to receive, which were meant simply to kill.

My Half-Life as a Dirty Bomb

I came to see cancer in a different way but at first I saw it very much in military terms. A mutation had established a beach head in the cells of my body. If I were to survive, the invasion had to be repelled, and two months into the process testosterone deprivation had softened cancer's position. Supply lines had been interrupted, driving advance forces back to the main base, and it was now time to hit cancer central with the full weight of the atomic arsenal.

But what did that mean really?

At first, when I checked out what X-rays did to my cells, it was like finding out what goes into hot dogs. There are some things you don't want to know, but that was the kind of attitude that had gotten me into this whole mess in the first place, the idea that I could avoid cancer by ignoring cancer.

Radiation is big business. You can't avoid it. There is no harmless dose, but there is a threshold value beyond which the chance of cell mutations quickly rises. Higher doses bring higher dangers, the more procedures you receive the greater your chance of developing mutated cells, and the effective total dose of radiation the typical American receives more than doubled, mostly due to increased use of high energy procedures such as CAT scans, between 1980 and 2006.

Of course, there is no such thing as a typical American.

Not when it comes to radiation. Reactions are cell specific; one study measuring skin damage found an 80 percent difference in sensitivity to radiation, another study on fibroblasts found tissue damage varied among a group of 41 patients by 350 percent. The take home lesson is that from one cell to the next the ability to withstand a given burst of radiation varies over a broad spectrum, and that variation isn't random.

There are reasons for it, simple reasons based on how radiation destroys cells. Some of it's genetic, some isn't. This is where both science and common sense say you can help yourself, even if you're only getting a chest X-ray, because based on published data "it is possible to develop a nontoxic, cost-effective mixture of antioxidants...that can provide biological protection against radiation damage in humans."

So, if a dirty bomb goes off in your neighborhood...

Take advantage of that monumental variation in cellular radiosensitivity. As a cancer patient, stack the odds in your favor. There's plenty you can do to limit both the metastasis that might kill you and side effects that might make you wish you were dead; this is particularly relevant when you've received enough radiation to kill a cockroach.

The amount of radiation a human body absorbs can be measured in units called *Gray*, after a British doctor named Gray. A typical curative total radiation dose over the course of cancer treatment averages maybe 60-80 Gray, yet a dose of only about 4.5 Gray will kill about half the people exposed to it within thirty days.

This is the $LD_{50\text{-}30}$, where LD is the lethal dose of radiation that kills 50 percent of a given population in thirty days. For humans, it's on the order of 4.5 Gray, goldfish 20 Gray, cockroaches 64 Gray, and shellfish about 200 Gray. The shielding power of clams is impressive, but it's nothing compared to Conan the Bacterium, the most radio-resistant animal life form on Earth so far encountered, which can withstand an instantaneous dose of 5,000 Gray with no discernable loss of viability.

As humans, the amount of radiation we receive during cancer treatment would be way more than enough to kill us but for two factors. First, curative levels of radiation are delivered to only a small part rather than the whole of the body. Second, total doses are *fractionated,* or spread out over time.

This is when it's time for an expert.

My situation was complicated by the fact that a fraction of my radiation would come from seeds planted directly into my prostate. The key here is spacing the seeds to avoid cold spots that might not kill the cancer and hot spots that might kill too much of me. The laws of electromagnetism determine this spacing, and the laws of spacing show the closest opening to the prostate is anal in nature. I expected my butt to hurt, but when I woke up after the seed implant operation I wondered why it was that my penis hurt worse.

Ah, the indignities.

I'm sure they told me but no way can you keep up with everything you hear. As long as you're out cold with your pants in the next room, standard operating procedure dictates a check for bladder cancer also, and the laws of spacing show that the closest opening to the bladder is the hole at the end of Mister Happy.

Just because two openings share the same underwear doesn't mean they both need be violated. That logic is far from absolute, but protocols are protocols, and Mister Happy was sore because he'd just had a camera shoved down his throat. Talk about invasive diagnostic procedures. My first urination later that night was like peeing screaming, bloody ground glass instead of the usual joyful water, so it was with mixed emotions the next morning that I viewed Doctor Seed's question:

"How do you feel?"

If there's one thing I've learned it's that whining gets you nowhere.

"Pretty good," I said.

Doctor Seed nodded, flipping through papers on a clipboard.

"Everything went well," he said. "A few things..."

The conversation was quite short. The inference was that at this point radiation and hormone deprivation would either work or it wouldn't work. Everything that could be done was being done, and Doctor Seed stood up behind his desk.

"One final thought," he said. "Do you take vitamin supplements?"

"Sometimes. When I think about it."

"Well," he said, "for the next couple of months you should avoid antioxidants like vitamin E. They can interfere with the effects of the radiation on the tumor."

The medical community is very much split on whether you should take antioxidants during radiation therapy. There's more on this later, but if you look at it from the point of the cell with an eye toward limiting metastasis and undesired side effects, it's hard to pick a time when it's more important that you eat antioxidants than during radiation. However, at the time, if Doctor Seed told me to do something, I did it.

"Sure," I said, "No problem."

I stood up, gingerly. It would be a long hobble to the airport, so Doctor Seed had plenty of time to walk over and hand me an official-looking embossed card.

"What's this?" I asked.

"In case you want to cross a border," he said. "Your seeds are emitting enough radiation to set off the sensitive instruments they use to detect terrorist smuggling."

I stopped dead in my limp. I flashed back to high school, and what I'd told the guidance counselor when she'd asked me what I thought I might be when I grew up, and how a dirty bomb wasn't any of them.

"That's a lot of radiation," I said.

Being a cancer doctor must be tough. Too many people don't get better, and Doctor Seed looked over at the rain in the window to avoid the tears in my eyes.

"Yes," he said. "It is."

Radioactivity is measured in half lives, the time it takes for half a given quantity of an unstable radioactive element to decay into a stable, unradioactive end-product. The half-life of my particular isotope is seventeen days, and convention says the effects of radiation become moot after five half lives, so for the purposes of my treatment I would be considered radiation free in eighty-five days.

On the other hand, no matter how many times you take half of a half you never get down to zero. As long as I lived, every so often, I'd be shooting off gamma rays. This matters because the effects of radiation are cumulative, and in a few months I would also undergo a second round of radiation, this time delivered externally to treat the area surrounding the prostate where it was so likely the cancer had already spread.

Regardless of the timing and dose at which external radiation is applied great strides have been made in the equipment in recent years. Modern machines are capable of delivering radiation with great accuracy and with intensity modulation from moment to moment, which helps focus more death on tumors and less on surrounding tissue. Unfortunately that wasn't the kind of machine I could afford.

There were better machines in other places but I didn't have the time or money to spend the couple months it would take to get radiated in any of those places. I was stuck with the nearest machine in the Montana hinterlands, and if the proton machine is akin to a precision laser, then the machine from which I received my daily dose of external radiation was more of a pirate's cannon loaded with rusty nails and shards of glass from broken bottles of rum.

You may think I'm kidding and I only wish I was.

On the second day of my treatment with external radiation, as I lay on a vinyl shelf in a cold concrete room in the basement of a hospital, naked but for a flimsy blue gown and wool socks, the X-ray machine, which when operating was as loud as a car crash, ground to a halt. The overhead florescent lights went black, and in the sudden deafening silence bare red bulbs began flashing on the walls.

It was all I could do not to get up and run.

"What!" I yelled. "What!"

The smiling X-Ray Lady was nonchalant as she ambled up.

"Oh, honey, don't y'all worry none," she said. "It's just the power."

The only illumination in the room came from the red flashing emergency lights and the technician in charge was telling me not to worry.

"'Just the power'...What do you mean, 'Just the power'?"

"Oh, honey," she replied, "It happens all the time."

Now there was some good news.

The X-Ray Lady overseeing my treatment was a "traveler," up from the Deep South with an accent to match. She'd been dishing out X-rays for more than thirty years, which meant she had experience with the antiquated relic of a linear accelerator that was being used to irradiate my body. The machine was enamel white, about half the size of a refrigerator, and mounted on a thick metallic arm that rotated the entire apparatus all the way around a narrow table upon which I lay.

During each daily treatment I received a stream of X-rays from the top, bottom, left, and right; one stop of the machine in each quadrant. At each stop X-Ray Lady would slide in a different shaped piece of lead with a cutout in the shape of my prostate and seminal vesicles at that angle. It is very much an archaic way of administering radiation, and each daily treatment began from the top, when a red laser from the machine was lined up with a small blue dot that had been tattooed on my abdomen.

This basic procedure was all that aligned my prostate with the X-rays, and there was no way to confirm continued proper alignment as the machine rotated around my body. That was entirely a function of my remaining motionless throughout the twenty or so minutes each treatment took, and that was on a good day.

On a bad day, I'd lay there until the machine started working again.

Over the course of my treatment the machine broke down at least once a week and usually more often than that. It always died in the middle of a dose, the clamor of the car crash suddenly just gone. And there I'd lay in the silence, so scared, my thin blue cotton gown soaked in chilling sweat, trying not to move.

Scrunch a bit this way and, when the power returned, I'd be frying my rectum instead of my prostate. Scrunch a tad the other way, now I'd be toasting my bladder. Take your pick, urine or feces, either way you don't want to burn a hole in the container.

That first day the power went out it was tough to talk around the lump in my throat, but I tried, slowly emphasizing each word so I wouldn't choke on it.

"If the power went out in the middle of a treatment...how do you know how much radiation you gave me?"

And how much more I'm supposed to get?

"Honey," said X-Ray Lady, "don't y'all worry none. The computer keeps track. We'll pick up right where we left off when the lights come back on."

A computer was in charge. Oh great.

We all know computers don't make mistakes.

Ionizing Radiation

There's a huge variation in the response of individual cells, both mutant and normal, to radiation. You want to stack the odds in your favor, to do what you can to help radiation kill cancer cells while preventing damage to healthy cells, and what you do is a function of the nature of the ionizing radiation with which you are bombarded.

Ionizing radiation has short wavelengths and high energy, so much energy that, when encountering an atom or molecule, these waves can blast electrons from their orbits. This creates ions, or charged particles that are in violation of the universal electric code that demands electrical neutrality.

In cells, electron-hungry ions are called free radicals, and they're hungry enough for electric neutrality that they can yank electrons right out of your molecules. This is a prime factor in aging, and it's much easier for free radicals to pry electrons from molecules of sugar-based DNA than from molecules of most fats and proteins.

DNA is among a select group of molecules that typically show the effects of cellular radiation first, and damage can happen directly or indirectly. Direct radiation hits on DNA are like something out of *Star Wars*, akin to vaporization, but DNA occupies only a tiny fraction of the total volume of the cell. Direct hits are rare and most damage to DNA from radiation accrues from free radicals created by indirect hits on the primary component of every cell: water.

Ionizing radiation breaks molecular bonds in water molecules (H_2O), creating positively charged hydrogen ions (H^+) and negatively charged hydroxyl ions (OH^-). This extremely unstable situation spawns reactions that create a variety of ever more potent electron thieves that have been implicated in many crimes against humanity, including wrinkling of the skin, liver disease, atherosclerosis, and Alzheimer's.

In this corner: "Free Radicals!"

"Boo. Hiss. Yuh bum, yuh."

And, in this corner: "Antioxidants!"

"Yay. Go get 'em, champ. Hooray."

You have ringside tickets to one of the fastest ongoing fights in the solar system, because free radicals are a normal by-product of the process of oxidation and respiration that fuels our cells. Free radicals are part of the price we pay for the energy it requires to be a higher life form and, as thieves go, free radicals are exceptionally quick. They pick your molecular pocket of electrons in mere nanoseconds.

As fast as free radicals are, antioxidants are faster. They can neutralize free radicals before damage is even done, but only if they show up for the fight. Healthy cells don't just need antioxidants; they need lots of antioxidants, particularly when being bombarded with ionizing radiation that creates abnormally high levels of free radicals.

What did you eat today?

As an example of the difference between eating processed foods and eating fruits and vegetables, consider a study that showed supplementation of beta carotene for a week prior to examinations involving diagnostic radiation significantly reduced X-ray induced radiation damage. Beta carotene is the chemical your body uses to make vitamin A, a potent antioxidant. Beta carotene is also the compound that is siphoned off and discarded when palm oil is fractionated into palm butter, and the chemical that when concentrated gives carrots their distinctive color.

When was the last time a doctor told you to eat carrots before an X-ray?

While I waited for radiation, they offered cookies and doughnuts.

Honestly, it's nuts. Sugar feeds the anaerobic nature of cancer. There's no doubt about this, just as there's no doubt antioxidants neutralize DNA-corrupting free radicals. So, the next time you pass by that tempting box of glazed and jelly doughnuts in the radiation ward...pass it by...it's just one more example of how you have to take charge of your own health care.

The amount of diagnostic radiation Americans receive increased 570 percent between 1980 and 2006 and continues to rise. Studies show a 1 to 3 percent increased risk of cancer as a result of these procedures, and procedures that use more radiation like barium enemas (now that sounds like fun) carry more risk. One to 3 percent isn't much, but it isn't negligible, especially if you're the one or three who gets it.

If you're getting zapped, why not stack the odds in your favor?

Supply your cells with lots and lots of antioxidants to attack the free radicals they are about to encounter. Load up on salads, take a high quality vitamin supplement. It only makes sense, and the amount of antioxidants your cells have to fight back against the free radicals created by ionizing radiation is certainly a factor in that huge variation in the response of individual cells to radiation.

You can and should send care packages to your cells, but, as fast as antioxidants are, they can't get every free radical. In humans, on an average day, even if you're not getting radiation for cancer, estimates of the number of daily DNA lesions free radicals impart range from one thousand to one million, *per cell.*

If this bothers you it shouldn't. It's just an indication of how adept you are—even if you've never picked up a hammer—at fixing things. The difference between a thousand and a million also indicates how much trouble you can stave off before it even happens by avoiding carcinogens and providing your cells with nutrients.

It's odd a molecule as critical as DNA was built around a backbone of sugar that is so easily dismantled by oxidation; one possible explanation for this fragility is that the organic chemistry of DNA that allowed cells to store information evolved long before the planet developed appreciable levels of free oxygen. DNA existed for billions of years before atmospheric oxygen levels rose significantly, at which point the single-celled organisms of the time were able to mount a defense against the challenge oxygen posed.

The solution—and this is the ongoing miracle of life— was to develop the genetic code that would whip up the fats and proteins that could cope with the problem. It was easier for life to resolve the oxygen predicament than to go back to square one and come up with a whole new system of chemical code that would store information, and cellular life developed defenses on two levels.

First, life used the power of the sun to create chemicals we call antioxidants that would react with and neutralize free radicals before they caused damage. Second, the miracle that is life evolved the genetic code to link the specific sequence of hundreds of amino acids into the complex proteins that are your DNA repair crews.

Repairs begin instantaneously and single-strand breaks—breaks in one side rail of the DNA ladder—are easy to mend. Repair molecules cut out the remaining pieces of a damaged nucleotide, insert a properly assembled nucleotide, and voilà, the DNA is again complete. It's like snapping together Legos. Single-strand breaks are typical of normal cellular operations and are easy to repair because the purchase order for the proper repair part is contained onsite across the ladder in the remaining DNA.

Double-strand breaks—which are breaks in both rails of the DNA ladder at or near the same location—are more difficult to restore. These breaks are more typical of the concentrated energies imparted by radiation, and to repair the damage the proper genetic sequence must be obtained from undamaged genetic material in another part of the nucleus. This information must be first sent for, and then relayed back to the site of the damage, and only then can complex repairs begin.

There's more chance of errors, but the repair of double-strand breaks is just one more task at which your cells excel. For instance, a 2002 study examined twenty-seven terminal cancer patients with lymph node metastases who received high (5 Gray) doses of radiation as palliative (non-curative) treatment for pain. Samples of the irradiated tissue were extracted at one, two, and three minutes, then analyzed for evidence of genetic reconstruction. The study concluded that even at these high levels of radiation, which would be expected to impart a high proportion of double-strand breaks, the half-life of DNA repair in these highly irradiated cells was less than five minutes.

Too bad they were cancer cells.

This same study, citing other studies, said that "there seems to be no significant difference in DNA repair between tumor and normal cells." Data from cells in dishes must be applied with caution to cells in humans, but, still, this was in stark contrast to the conventional wisdom on which I'd based my decision to get radiation, which was that undifferentiated cancer cells are less likely to be able to repair radiation damage, and therefore more likely to die than normal cells.

Conventional wisdom also holds cancer cells are more likely to sustain fatal damage from radiation than healthy cells. This idea has roots in the dual premise that cancer cells tend to reproduce more quickly than normal cells, and that actively dividing cells are more susceptible to radiation than cells that are at "rest."

Actually, while biologists describe cells that aren't actively dividing as "resting," these cells are doing anything but resting. These cells are working, constantly sending and receiving messages, each cell unceasingly cranking out its own particular blend of the many fats and proteins necessary to keep your body alive.

During this phase, the DNA is loosely spread around the nucleus like unspooled thread, which makes the genetic code readily accessible so the reactions of life can proceed. The term for this diffused DNA is *chromatin,* and the thinly dispersed chromatin is less susceptible to radiation damage because it does not make a centralized target and because repair molecules can be promptly dispatched to damaged DNA.

DNA is more concentrated in cells that are actively dividing. The process of cell division includes four distinct phases of DNA activity and typically lasts a couple of days overall, and each phase is more or less susceptible to radiation damage. The cell is most susceptible during the last phase, the thirty to sixty minutes of mitosis, when the cell is actually dividing from one cell into two, and the DNA is packed in a dense rod of coils within coils within coils.

This is when the DNA is arranged in the classic X-shape of chromosomes, and the tightly coiled molecule is more likely to take fatal hits from incoming radiation for a couple of reasons. First, the densely packed molecule makes a solid target that is more likely to be hit by incoming radiation. Second, a direct hit on coils within coils within coils of DNA is likely to take out more genetic material at once, and as that damage accumulates it quickly becomes impossible to repair.

THE HUMAN HARD DRIVE

Nucleotide, the basic building block of DNA

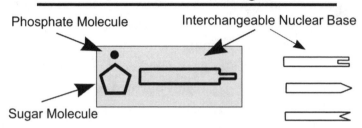

Phosphate Molecule

Interchangeable Nuclear Base

Sugar Molecule

Your DNA is a long chain of "nucleotides" which lock together like Legos. Three Legos in a row spell the code for a particular amino acid, hundreds of Legos in a row amount to the recipes your cells follow to build the many proteins of which you are made.

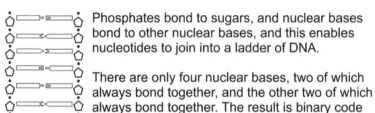

Phosphates bond to sugars, and nuclear bases bond to other nuclear bases, and this enables nucleotides to join into a ladder of DNA.

There are only four nuclear bases, two of which always bond together, and the other two of which always bond together. The result is binary code with backup, and it's a good thing life is better at backup than I am, or we'd have died out long ago.

←— Single Strand Break

Breaks to one side rail of DNA are easy to repair because only one nucleotide can fit into the open space...your cells know exactly what to do.

←— Double Strand Break

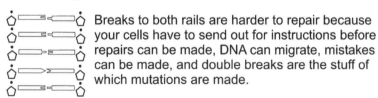

Breaks to both rails are harder to repair because your cells have to send out for instructions before repairs can be made, DNA can migrate, mistakes can be made, and double breaks are the stuff of which mutations are made.

It's the difference between dropping an atomic bomb in the middle of the ocean or the middle of a city; bombs in the city do more damage to important infrastructure. If you radiate a cancer cell in the process of mitosis, mission accomplished. If you radiate a healthy cell in the process of mitosis, well, in the Army they call it friendly fire, but there's nothing friendly about it.

Tumors aren't solid masses of cancer cells. They're heterogeneous jumbles of normal cells, highly mutated cells, and somewhat mutated cells surrounded by healthy cells in healthy tissue. When it comes to these cells, radiation does not play favorites, it nukes them all.

When radiation hits a healthy cell the hope is that the cell can repair whatever damage has accrued and remain healthy. If the cell can't fix itself, plan B is that the cell will kill itself for the common good. If the cell doesn't die, and instead passes corrupted genetic material down to daughter cells, then you have the makings of more cancer instead of less. This is the mutagenic nature of radiation, and is a major limitation on the effectiveness of radiation as a cancer treatment.

It's a crap shoot, and the game has long been run according to the principles of what sounds more like a Cajun zydeco band than a guiding light of radiotherapy. This is the 1906 Law of Bergonie and Tribondeau, named after the two French scientists who came up with it, which postulates that cells displaying the following three characteristics will be more sensitive to the effects of radiation:

1) Cells that are rapidly dividing.
2) Cells that have a long dividing future ahead of them.
3) Cells that are of an unspecialized type.

This is where the idea came from that cancer cells would be more likely to die from radiation than healthy cells, but in practical usage the law has become more of a rule of thumb. The bottom line is that, given what we now know, for many reasons, the specific kind and amount of damage a given animal cell will sustain when exposed to a given amount of radiation cannot be predicted with accuracy.

This is as true of cancer cells as it is of normal cells. Even so, you would think that the most fundamental check on Bergonie and Tribondeau would begin with Petri dishes full of cells, some cancerous, some normal. These cultures would then be irradiated, and then examined to see how cancer cells fared as opposed to healthy cells.

This is a very simple experiment, and simple experiments tend to produce the data that is the least misleading. You'd think this utterly basic research would have been performed many times in many ways, but that wasn't so, at least with prostate cells.

A sweeping 2005 review out of Stanford University, summarizing research of in vitro prostate cell cultures and citing nearly 250 papers, stated that since "radiotherapy is a widely used treatment option for men with prostate cancer, it is surprising that relatively little has been done to investigate radiation sensitivity and response of primary cultures." In fact, this review found only two studies in which the relative effect of radiation on cancerous versus normal cells was examined.

The first, a 2003 study at the Department of Medical Biophysics in the University of Toronto, compared the effects of radiation on two lines of healthy prostate cells and four lines of malignant cells. Radiation was applied at 2 Gray to simulate a dose typical of fractionated radiation therapy. Cell survival following radiation was much greater in all four lines of cancer cells, and ranged from 5 percent survival for one healthy prostate cell line to 55 percent survival for one line of prostate cancer cells, "suggesting that malignant prostate cells are more radio-resistant than normal prostate cells, for this series."

WHAT!!!

For every cancer cell destroyed by radiation as many as ten healthy cells could be dying. That's no suggestion, that's a declaration, and I had a vested interest in every one of those healthy rectal, bladder, blood, and nerve cells surrounding my prostate.

Again, this was utterly contrary to the conventional wisdom that cancer cells are more easily killed by radiation than normal cells. In fact, the latest research shows that the anaerobic nature of cancer instigates chemical reactions that defend cancer cells from radiation in ways that normal cells can't. When it comes to resisting radiation, cancer is more like Superman than Clark Kent, so it's a good thing we have some kryptonite.

The second study cited in the Stanford review of the effects of radiation on prostate cells was published in 2003 in the *British Journal of Cancer*, and examined the potentially synergistic effects of varying amounts of ionizing radiation in combination with varying amounts of two vitamin D derivatives. Results were dose dependent for both the amounts of radiation and vitamin D applied to the cell cultures, and benefits were muted at high levels of radiation and high concentrations of vitamin D.

Again, too much of anything is too much for you.

Results in this experiment were measured by the combination index, an overall measure of culture survival, where an index of 1.0 was representative of cell survival in control cultures. Beneficial interaction was highest at radiation doses of 1 Gray (about half the daily dose in typical fractionated radiotherapy) and moderate concentrations of calcitriol (the active metabolite of vitamin D). The combination index for this treatment regimen indicated an overall survival of .53 for cancer cells, and an overall survival of 1.60 for normal cells.

This is the ultimate good news: benign concentrations of vitamin D rendered prostate cancer cells nearly 50 percent more susceptible to death by radiation, and healthy prostate cells 60 percent less susceptible. The study concluded that the presence of calcitriol, at concentrations that can be feasibly reached in the human body, allowed for a 2.4 times lower dose of radiation to obtain the same therapeutic effect.

If this were an experiment on humans, it's one for which I would have volunteered. It's a very different approach than most of what I read, which was that since radiation is limited in its ability to kill cancer cells, the solution is to apply more radiation to kill cancer cells. To me, this makes sense in the same way that while more and more radiation will certainly destroy your cancer, so will jumping off an ever-higher cliff.

Don't forget when considering the study on radiation and vitamin D that cells in humans act differently than cells in a laboratory dish. At the same time, this is not isolated evidence. As another example of the synergistic effects of antioxidants and radiation, consider the traditional Ayurvedic herbal medicine Triphala.

Triphala, meaning "three fruits," is a combination of three plants, all of which have been shown to contain chemicals that function as potent antioxidants. Several different studies have shown Triphala induces death in cancer cells while sparing healthy cells, and that at doses typical of fractionated radiotherapy it renders cancer cells more susceptible to death by radiation and healthy cells less susceptible.

But wait, there's more.

The sugar molecules in the DNA backbone are easily attacked by the free radicals created by ionizing radiation, but so are the electron-dangling polyunsaturated fatty acids found in the phospholipids of the cell membrane. Again, advantage cancer, because, as stated in a 2005 paper in the *Journal of Cancer Research Therapy*, "Cancer cell membranes are known to be deficient in polyunsaturated fatty acids, which renders them radio-resistant."

Better reach for the kryptonite.

The deficiency in polyunsaturated fatty acids is an advantage you can negate. Begin your day with a flax oil smoothie. Many lines of evidence from many reputable institutions indicate that restoring levels of polyunsaturated fatty acids to your cell membranes makes those cells less likely to become cancerous, more likely to destroy themselves if cancerous, and more likely to die by radiation when cancerous.

The same goes for studies on antioxidants, including vitamins A, D, and E, and Triphala. It isn't just one thing, it's everything. Grab the advantage of that huge variation in the response of all cells, both mutant and normal, to radiation. Flood a cancer cell membrane with highly unsaturated fatty acids and that cell is more likely to burst in the presence of ionizing radiation. Flood healthy cells with antioxidants and they are more likely to survive an onslaught of free radicals without damage.

There are no magic bullets, and I can't tell you what to do. Plenty of doctors would cite plenty of studies against the idea of taking antioxidants during radiation. All I can do is tell you what worked for me, and why I think it worked, and again we come back to the common theme of oxygen and the energy it provides.

It's a different way of looking at how to best rid your body of cancer. Treat cause, not symptom, and according to this theory the cause of mutated cells is oxidative stress that creates the symptom of damaged DNA. This is not a wild-eyed, crazy idea. The notion that oxidative stress is fundamental to the nature of a cancer cell is nothing new, dating back to the 1920s and Nobel Prize winning research on the nature of respiration by a German named Otto Warburg.

The Warburg Effect

As I researched this book the name Otto Warburg kept popping up in the company of unlikely scientific bedfellows. For instance, Johanna Budwig based her diet on research that stemmed from Warburg's findings, while mainstream cutting edge 2008 scientific papers on the nature of hypoxia and cancer also cited Warburg's research.

Who, I wondered, was this guy?

Just, it seems, another stone-cold genius.

Warburg was born to a Christian mother and a Jewish father in Germany in 1883. At the age of thirty, with a doctorate in chemistry and a medical degree already under his belt, he was awarded his own laboratory at the Kaiser Wilhelm Institute. His early research on how cell growth affected oxygen consumption was interrupted by a stint in the Prussian cavalry in World War I, where he carried not only a pistol but a medieval lance. He was wounded on the Russian front, and finally returned to his laboratory in 1918 at the urgings of Albert Einstein.

Warburg was nominated for a Nobel Prize in 1927 for work on the metabolism of cancer cells, research that provided a foundation for study of the nature of respiration as a whole. The question Warburg was trying to answer, in its simplest terms, begins with a bowl of sugar. That sugar, sitting at room temperature on a table, does not react to produce energy. Yet that same sugar, in living cells at the same temperature, does react to produce energy. Otto Warburg set out to solve this puzzle of fundamental cellular mechanics, and the answer would win him the Nobel Prize for Physiology in 1931.

At the time, it had been known for over a century that certain metals acting as catalysts accelerated the rate at which inorganic chemical reactions occurred. Warburg hypothesized these inorganic processes somehow related to the organic world, yet the technology of the time was simply unable to separate out the infinitesimal concentration of any such chemicals from the cells to which those chemicals were so firmly bound.

Warburg devised techniques and equipment that allowed for indirect methods of measurement. A series of experiments eventually demonstrated that iron was the active ingredient in the process Warburg described as "cellular respiration," yet exact chemical descriptions of the enzyme iron-oxygenase would have to await the advent of X-ray crystallography techniques decades later. Herr Warburg was able to transcend the technology of the time, and isolate iron as a catalyst in the energetic reactions of human cells based, in part, on his observations of a fundamental difference in the metabolism of cancer cells and healthy cells.

The nature of cancer was to remain a focus of Warburg's formidable research career. As one estimate of his significance in this field consider that Warburg, a Jew, was allowed (forced) to maintain his laboratory in Germany throughout World War II, in part (it is speculated) because of Hitler's fear of this disease. Decades of follow-up research into the fundamental chemistries of the energies of life led Doctor Warburg to conclude, in 1966, at a speech he delivered to a gathering of Nobel Laureates that:

Cancer, above all other diseases, has countless secondary causes...but only one prime cause...the replacement of the respiration of oxygen in normal body cells by a fermentation of sugar. From the standpoint of the physics and chemistry of life this difference between normal and cancer cells is so great that one can scarcely picture a greater difference. Oxygen gas...is dethroned in the cancer cells and replaced by an energy yielding reaction of the lowest living forms, namely, a fermentation of glucose.

The lowest living forms include, aside from fishing guides at two in the morning, yeast. There are many species of yeast and many fermentation reactions, but in one familiar example brewer's yeast processes one molecule of glucose into two molecules of ethanol, two molecules of carbon dioxide, and two molecules of energy in the form of adenosine tri-phosphate (ATP), a complex protein that uses phosphate bonds to first store energy in the form of electrons, and then deliver that energy on demand to the cellular components that require it.

ATP is the energetic currency of life. It's like money. You need it to live well, you either have it or you don't, and it takes work to get. The shortcoming of fermentation is that while it does provide cells with energy, it leaves most of the money on the table.

Brewer's yeast leaves that money in the form of ethanol, a highly energetic molecule that is used to fuel both automobiles and New Year's Eve parties. Cells needed a key to get at that locked up energy, and that key was electron-starved oxygen atoms that drove the process that became known as respiration. The relatively low energy of fermentation is as familiar as the bubbles in a vat of brewing beer; the highly energetic reaction of respiration is a whole different ballgame, and as familiar as fire.

Respiration releases much more energy than fermentation because respiration picks up where fermentation leaves off. Your cells
use the potential energy stored in oxygen to release the potential
energy stored in the by-products of fermentation in what amounts
to a veritable swap-meet of electrons. Buyers come, sellers go,
step-by-step and enzyme-by-enzyme as complex molecules are
reduced to simpler molecules.

The next time you're on *Jeopardy* you can tell them this is the
Krebs cycle, and the end result of all this electron swapping is that
a single molecule of glucose can react with six molecules of oxygen
to yield six molecules of carbon dioxide, six molecules of water,
and thirty-eight molecules of stored energy in the form of ATP.

If this was a high school football game the energy score would be:
Respiration: 38.
Fermentation: 2.

It's not even close, and this respiration-induced ATP energy sur-
feit makes the high degree of differentiation typical of human cells
possible. The disadvantages of respiration include that it is slower
than fermentation and it requires an excess of free oxygen. When
straining human cells—such as the muscles in your legs when running from a wolf—demand oxygen at rates faster than is being supplied by your blood then your cells can turn to fermentation as a
short term answer.

A little extra energy might be the difference between eating and
being eaten, but in human cells the by-product of fermentation is
lactic acid. The acidic environment created by fermentation impairs the chemical reactions of respiration, and muscles under
strain can run on the energy of fermentation for only so long before the acid build-up must be reversed. You have to stop to catch
your breath, and absorb some oxygen, which will break down the
lactic acid, and absorb some more oxygen, which will restore respiration and normal cellular energy balances.

Our cells are hard-wired to turn to fermentation for energy production when necessary, but only on a short term basis. When fermentation becomes chronic—such as when trans fats impede the normal flow of oxygen through the plasma cell membrane—then our cells quickly become deprived of the energy necessary for normal operations. And when our cells can't operate normally, they can just as quickly become abnormal.

In the simplest of terms it is this fundamental difference between the relative energies produced by oxidation and fermentation that Otto Warburg saw as the cause of cancer. In his view all cancer cells consistently derive some portion of their energy requirements through fermentation, and therefore do not have enough energy to go around. It is a simple observation with profound implications, including the fact that you don't need an HMO to change the levels of usable oxygen in your cells.

Suffice it to say good scientists do not necessarily make good writers. In general, researching this book was an ordeal of wading through sentences that weren't sentences, misleading double negatives, and waffling equivocation, the whole of it bobbing in an alphabet soup of coded acronyms. In contrast, Warburg's succinct prose was like a breath of fresh air after eight hours in an airplane.

In science, good experimental technique is paramount, and the speech honoring Warburg at his Nobel acceptance ceremony in 1931 cited him for "rare perfection in the art of exact measurement." Warburg details his techniques like recipes in a cookbook for the proper care and feeding of laboratory cancer, and summarizes much of his early research in a 1927 paper on "The Metabolism of Tumors in the Body."

At the time nobody knew what they would find; what Warburg and others found was that tumors in both animals and humans used up large amounts of glucose and produced large amounts of lactic acid. As an example of how early scientists figured this out, in one early experiment a tumor was implanted into one wing of an unlucky chicken.

After the tumor was allowed to take root, samples of blood were drawn from both wings; in 100 cubic centimeters of blood there were 23 milligrams less glucose and 16 milligrams more lactic acid in the tumor wing. A similar experiment was then performed on a human with a tumor in one forearm; again blood drawn from the forearm with the tumor showed significantly more lactic acid and significantly less glucose. The process of fermentation requires glucose and produces lactic acid. Warburg attributed the drop in glucose and rise in lactic acid levels to the fact that those tumors were deriving some portion of their total energy requirements via fermentation.

In follow-up experiments to test the theory, levels of lactic acid and glucose were measured in samples of blood drawn above and below normal tissue, and above and below tumors. Levels of lactic acid within limits of experimental error either decreased or remained the same above and below normal tissue, a zero (0) amount of change, which you would expect of resting tissue obtaining all its energy via respiration. Levels of lactic acid below the tumors, on the other hand, increased in every instance, by an average of 46 milligrams in 100 cubic centimeters of blood.

Mathematically, this percentage increase in lactic acid between tumors and healthy tissue is so large it can't be expressed. It would be 46 divided by 0, but you can't divide by 0 since the result is infinity, an impossible answer.

These huge differences in blood lactic acid levels are extremely unlikely to be the result of anything but fermentation. There is no need to fabricate complex theories involving dozens of messenger proteins to explain the results and, crucially, because this is a factor every cancer patient can and should control, blood glucose levels also varied significantly between normal and cancerous tissues.

Warburg found that on average normal tissue took 2-16 milligrams of glucose from 100 cubic centimeters of blood, while tumors took an average of 70 milligrams of glucose from the blood. This difference, while not infinite, is still vast, on the order of hundreds of percent. Cancer loves sugar, but even undifferentiated cancer cells can't survive solely on the energy of fermentation indefinitely.

Early experiments showed that different tumors survived in the absence of oxygen in serums containing glucose for varying lengths of time, generally about one to three days. After that time the energy of fermentation wasn't sufficient to sustain the cancer cells. Free oxygen was necessary to provide the additional energy the cells needed to survive, and further experiments (both in vivo and in vitro) showed that most cancer cells, when deprived of both oxygen and glucose, died in about four hours.

Now there's a cure for cancer.

Or is it?

Deprive tissues of both glucose and oxygen for four hours and cancer cells will die; unfortunately, so will normal cells. Deprive tissues of oxygen and normal cells will die or mutate from lack of energy, while cancer cells survive through fermentation. On the positive side, if you deprive tissues of glucose, then cancer cells are most affected.

Somewhere in that medley of cause and effect Doctor Warburg hoped to find a cure to cancer by controlling levels of oxygen and glucose. He admitted the prospects were bleak, yet saw hope since "the resistance of single tumor cells is not to be compared with that of single normal cells, but rather the tumor as a whole with the organism as a whole. An overpopulated city is more sensitive to stoppage of food supply than a normally populated city, even when the inhabitants can all endure hunger alike."

Warburg, in other research, had shown that tumors generally demand more glucose than the blood supplies at normal concentrations. Therefore, he reasoned, the front half of a tumor—the part of the tumor that received the blood first—could exist on glucose alone (for a while), but there wouldn't be sufficient glucose to supply all the fermentation needs of the back half of the tumor. In the absence of the large amounts of glucose that fermentation demands the back half of the tumor would require oxygen to survive, and Warburg theorized that drastically reducing the oxygen supply while limiting available glucose might kill the back half of the tumor.

Killing half a tumor is a big step in the right direction and the experiment to test this hypothesis was simple. Rats with implanted tumors, with regular glucose levels in their blood, were placed in an airtight container in which the oxygen concentration was reduced to 5 percent by volume (as opposed to the normal 20 percent). A dash of ammonia was added to prevent acidosis in the rats, and Warburg found after several hours "the anticipated effect was achieved, but was far greater than expected."

Most of the tumor cells had been killed off, both front and back, "with only a thin outer shell showing normal metabolism." Warburg explained this result by the fact that once the back half of the tumor was destroyed, the capillary cells that supplied it were also destroyed, thus blocking the flow of blood, and stopping the supply in the front half of the tumor in the same manner that a lake backs up upstream of a dam.

"At first it seems paradoxical that cells which can live by fermentation can be killed off by want of oxygen," he said, "but there is really no contradiction here. Yeast cells, as well as tumor cells, can be killed through want of oxygen; in both cases only when the sugar required for fermentation is lacking."

The take-home lesson is that maybe you don't want to take that candy home.

Warburg next wondered why healthy cells might embrace fermentation in the first place. Oxygen deficits were an obvious potential cause, and to test this idea embryonic mouse cells were grown in vitro in the presence of varying amounts of oxygen. The cells grown in normal oxygen levels developed normally, but when oxygen pressures dropped to about 65 percent of normal the developing mouse embryos displayed fermentation as quickly as the second cell division, and these cells retained their characteristic fermentation even when re-exposed to an oxygen-rich environment.

In another experiment involving indirect methods tetanus spores were injected into healthy mice, and into mice with implanted tumors. Tetanus can germinate only at very low oxygen pressures and did not affect healthy mice. Mice with tumors sickened with tetanus, and again the evidence associated tumors with low oxygen levels.

Years of research led Warburg to conclude that "During the cancer development the oxygen respiration always fails, fermentation appears, and highly differentiated cells are transformed to fermenting anaerobes, which have lost all their body functions and retain only the now useless property of growth. Thus, when respiration disappears, life does not disappear, but the meaning of life disappears, and what remains are growing machines that destroy the body in which they grow."

For the next four decades, in a distinguished research career as director of the prestigious Max Planck Institute for Cell Physiology, Warburg pushed his theory that cancer is caused by cellular energy imbalances due to faulty respiration. To announce that you have found the cause of cancer, even for a Nobel laureate, is a bold claim, and Warburg took it personally when his theories were rejected by a medical community that focused decades of research dollars instead on viral or genetic causes of cancer.

Among other poetic insults, Warburg referred to his colleagues as prophets of agnosticism who had relapsed into the bygone times of medicine and caused millions of unnecessary deaths. As you can imagine, this did not endear Warburg to his peers, and over time he was increasingly dismissed as just another wild-eyed heretic, particularly as he applied the conclusions of his research to the habits of his personal life.

Warburg found the B vitamins and iron both play a crucial role in the process of respiration, and he went so far as to publicly proclaim that including these substances in the everyday diet could stave off cancer. Worse, as the years passed, he favored bread baked from wheat grown organically on his own land. His fanaticism was confirmed when it became known that, when in a restaurant, he would pay full price for a cup of tea, and then order only hot water, into which he would dunk his own bag of tea procured from sources he trusted.

That's pretty crazy all right.

During the last twenty years of his life, at a time when a lot of people will settle for working up a good drool, Warburg published a remarkable 178 scientific papers. He is said to have been physically fit and mentally active until the age of 85, when he was thrown from a horse and broke his leg, an injury from which he never fully recovered. Warburg died two years later in 1970, which he probably regretted, because forty years later he would have taken a great deal of pleasure in telling the prophets of agnosticism *"ich habe das schon gesacht,"* which is more or less German for "I told you so."

Hypoxia

The *Dictionary of Scientific Biography* ranks Otto Warburg as the greatest biochemist of all time by virtue of the number and magnitude of his discoveries. His is an astonishing body of work, and, when asked why his theories on the cause and cure of cancer were never fully embraced by his fellow scientists, Warburg liked to quote the physicist Max Planck, who said:

> A new scientific truth is often accepted, not as a result of opponents being convinced and declaring themselves won over, but rather by the opponents dying off, and the oncoming generation of scientists becoming familiar with the truth right from the start.

Well, the opponents are dying off, and a new generation of scientists is coming along. As the twenty-first century unravels, researchers are coming full circle back to Warburg's theories in a wealth of experiments designed to document the specific effects of *hypoxia* on the initiation, growth, and metastasis of cancer.

Hypoxia is essentially a state of "below normal" oxygen pressure in a given tissue. The higher the pressure of a gas the higher it pushes a column of mercury in a tube; most tissues run at oxygen pressures of about 20 millimeters of mercury. When the average partial pressure of oxygen dips below about 10 millimeters a cell gets worried for its life, and reacts to the dangerous situation by increasing the concentration of a molecule named hypoxia-inducible factor 1 (HIF-1).

I know what you're thinking.

Catchy name.

The messenger protein HIF-1 is a complex molecule that is highly conserved throughout the oxygen breathing cellular kingdom, and arranged in a configuration that can act directly on certain genes in the DNA with instructions to increase their activity. No need for a go-between. Something is wrong, seriously wrong. There isn't enough oxygen, and HIF-1 directly instructs the DNA to send messages that cause cancer cells to take several distinct actions—all bad for you, and all good for the cancer.

First, HIF-1 throws the switch that turns the cell from aerobic to anaerobic respiration, allowing cancer cells to survive through fermentation in conditions of low oxygen that would kill or mutate normal cells. Second, the cell is sentient enough to know that even though oxygen levels are low locally, they might be higher elsewhere.

It's all about survival, and HIF-1 also instructs the DNA to issue chemical orders that override the chemical messages that instruct specialized cells to bind together as tissues and organs. Prostate cells no longer receive the message to clump with other prostate cells, hit the lymph in search of oxygen, and generally lodge in the bones. Mutated breast cells no longer content with their heavenly lot in life tend to head off toward the liver, but no cancer cell is particular about where it ends up.

HIF-1 is like a mandate to metastasize, but it also triggers powerful survival mechanisms in the cancer cells that stay at home. Among the worst is a call for vascular endothelial growth factor

(VEGF), which in turn stimulates the production of new blood vessels to supply the missing oxygen, which in turn stimulates the tumor to grow. The growth of new blood vessels is called angiogenesis, and when cancer gets its own nutrient-rich supply of blood it is often the beginning of the end.

Until that blood arrives, the conditions of low oxygen instigate the production of chemical messengers that tell the cell to conserve energy by curtailing the production of normal proteins and fats. The hypoxic cancer cell goes into survival mode, and many studies show that this includes chemical instructions to put reproduction on hold until conditions improve. It's what you would expect, and a slowly dividing cancer cell would be a good thing, except traditional chemotherapy and radiotherapy are based on the idea that cancer cells reproduce more quickly than healthy cells.

Cells in survival mode are better able to fight off a variety of threats, including *cytotoxins,* the "cell-poisons" used in chemotherapy. Among other things, studies show hypoxia preferentially defends tumor cells from the effects of chemotherapy by reducing concentrations of cytotoxins within the cell, by reducing the effects of the cytotoxin that is there, and by increasing the chemical synthesis of proteins from the multi-drug resistance family that is a cell's normal defense against cytotoxins.

In other words, hypoxic cancerous cells employ your body's own natural defenses to their own mutated ends, and it works against radiation too.

When oxygen levels drop, cancer cells can approach a hibernation-like state, and in vitro studies show radiation is three times less likely to kill poorly oxygenated cells as opposed to well oxygenated cells. Other studies show that when hibernating cells put reproduction on hold the cancer cells are less susceptible to ionizing radiation that acts most effectively on clumped DNA during actual mitosis.

All that, from a simple lack of oxygen.

It kind of takes your breath away, doesn't it?

It did mine.

Low levels of oxygen cause high levels of HIF-1, which encourages unchecked cellular growth, cellular dedifferentiation, fermentation, angiogenesis, and metastasis. Everything cancer is, HIF-1 promotes by acting directly on DNA. If a lack of oxygen doesn't cause cancer, especially from the practical standpoint of how we as patients might improve our treatment outcomes, the distinction is so fine as to be moot.

But wait, there's more.

Under hypoxic conditions the processes of life can slow to the point that HIF-1 is preserved for future use in spore-like stress granules. These granules are programmed to open when oxygen levels again rise, and oxygen levels are rising and falling constantly in a typical tumor. Studies show oxygen concentrations in tumors are double-cyclical, a cycle within a cycle, each cycle with a unique frequency. In the shorter cycle oxygen levels rise and fall in smooth waves a couple times an hour, while the longer cycle is measured in hours or days and is superimposed on the shorter cycle in the same way the rise and fall of the tide controls the over-all height of individual ocean waves.

This cycle within a cycle, think qi.

A tumor isn't a solid mass of cancer cells. It's yin and yang, a mish-mash of healthy and unhealthy cells all grabbing at the available oxygen, which comes in waves. Studies show cancer preferentially evolves in this sea of constant change as opposed to stable chronic hypoxia, and when healthy cells die, say through apoptosis due to sensing an impending mutation, the oxygen that up-until-now healthy cell had been consuming becomes available for other cells to use.

Nearby cancer cells that have been laying semi-dormant waiting for oxygen can rumble to life. The HIF-1 laden stress capsules rupture, sending all the wrong signals, and starting the cycle all over again. This is the great advantage that cancer has. It's a mutation that is still mutating and as it mutates in hypoxic conditions it can evolve defenses against hypoxia in ways that normal cells can't.

Now let's add a dash of ionizing radiation to the mix.

The radiation creates free radicals, and too much oxygen in the form of free radicals is just as bad as too little oxygen in the form of hypoxia. The cell is under attack either way, and responds to both threats by producing HIF-1. It's a double whammy, and the high levels of electron scavenging free radicals created by ionizing radiation have the effect of stabilizing HIF-1 in hypoxic cells at high concentrations.

High levels of stabilized HIF-1 help hypoxic cancer cells fight the effects of radiation, and radiation causes high levels of stabilized HIF-1. The radioactive emperor has no clothes, only this monarch glows in the dark. Rather than calling the radioactive emperor on his lack of attire once and for all, a great deal of money is being spent on studies seeking chemicals that would effectively dress the radioactive emperor for dinner.

M-m-m, roast cancer cells.

The idea is that since radiation stabilizes HIF-1 levels, which in turn trigger a cascade of chemical messengers that promote the growth of cancer, it might in turn be possible to interfere with these chemical messengers so as to improve the effectiveness of radiation. The idea is logical, but if you're looking for a simple solution, this isn't it.

Our chemical messengers talk back and forth so much that it is difficult to control them. Block one pathway, they slip down another. HIF-1 is a cell's 9-1-1 call for emergency help. It's a big deal.

Things are seriously wrong. You better stop the call before it's made, because once it goes out, there is no stopping it, not really.

As an example, consider a cancerous cell as a burning house. Your goal is to burn down that house, so you chemically block the ability of that cell to call for the fire department. The emergency 9-1-1 call still goes out, just not to the fire department. Within minutes several police units, an emergency rescue crew, and the coroner all arrive at the scene of the fire. They look around.

"Where's the fire department?" they ask.

"Somebody get on the phone, and hurry."

The call goes out, and the fire department arrives. The cancer cell lives on and, in real cells, the communication potential is far greater than this simple example. Scientists have so far discovered three hypoxia-inducible factors, each of which is a potential 9-1-1 call, all proteins highly conserved throughout the kingdom of cells, and all of which trigger a cascade in the Pony Express system of chemical messengers that quickly swells from a trickle to a river of cross-talk.

Investigating this cascade of chemicals is interesting but expensive, and seems as unlikely to cure cancer as it is to raise your insurance rates. In trying to somehow make sense of this inchoate madness I can't tell you what to do, all I can do is tell you what I did, which was to again apply the premise that simple solutions are best because they're the least likely to be wrong.

Aristotle, in the tradition of the Greek philosophers, was a thinker in many fields. He had a theory on the origin of life; he also had theories on the nature of logic in the form of summarizing axioms. We take this kind of deductive reasoning for granted now but somebody had to think of it first, and one of Aristotle's enduring contributions to thinking came in the form of two premises and a conclusion:

Premise: All Greeks are men.

Premise: All men are mortal.

Conclusion: All Greeks are mortal.

HIF-1 promotes the initiation, growth, and metastasis of cancer. If our goal is to limit the production of this protein we might begin with two facts on which nearly all researchers agree, and apply Aristotelian logic as follows:

Premise: HIF-1 is produced in low oxygen environments.

Premise: HIF-1 is sustained in high free radical environments.

Conclusion: Dude, eat your vegetables and flaxseed oil.

Oxygenate your cells by providing them with highly unsaturated fatty acids that help build permeable plasma cell membranes. Arm your cells with the antioxidants they need to fight off the free radicals. Control levels of HIF-1 by controlling the production cues. It may not cure the cancer, but then again, it might.

Oxygen has to be carried to cells before it can get into cells, and since anemic blood carries oxygen poorly, it's no surprise anemia is common in cancer patients. Anemia is a deficiency in red blood cells and/or iron-rich hemoglobin, and low hemoglobin levels have been associated with increased tumor growth and decreased survival for many kinds of cancers. Statistics show anemics have much poorer cancer treatment outcomes, and, unfortunately, chemotherapeutic cytotoxins are particularly hard on rapidly reproducing red blood cells.

Chemotherapy-induced anemia has been routinely treated with very expensive FDA approved drugs that promote the growth of red blood cells. Regrettably, a 2009 paper that examined fifty-two clinical trials involving over twelve thousand patients found these drugs result in about a 16 percent increase in the risk of serious adverse coronary-related events, including death. That's one side effect; the second is increased insurance rates to cover attorney's fees in the tort suit that is probably impending. Our health system is so broken that it sometimes seems like the only way to fix it is to move to Canada, but the point isn't that we as patients should sit back and wring our hands.

The point is that we have to take matters into our own hands.

Highly profitable FDA approved drugs aren't the only way to add oxygen-carrying iron to your blood. Strict vegetarians beware: meat is a good source of an easily absorbed form of iron. A less easily absorbed form of iron is concentrated in beans, grains, and green leafy vegetables; absorption of this form of iron is enhanced when eaten along with vitamin C, and discouraged by the tannins in coffee and tea.

When you provide your blood with the raw materials it needs to carry oxygen, and your cells with the raw materials they need to absorb that oxygen, then you've gone a long way toward dealing with the prime causes of cellular oxygen deficits.

But what about the symptom?

"Hm-m-m..." you might be thinking, "that's easy enough."

Many studies show oxygenated cancer cells are more likely to be destroyed by radiation, so perhaps you're wondering what would happen if you just sucked at some oxygen while you were being radiated. Would that help?

A few studies have tested the effects of radiation on patients who breathed oxygen from tanks while receiving their radiation. One such 1995 experiment showed that breathing pure oxygen at normal pressures for fifteen or twenty minutes during the administration of radiation for head and neck cancer raised the three-year survival rate from 2 percent to 19 percent. On the other hand results with hyperbaric oxygen chambers, which can raise blood oxygen levels 2000 percent, have been inconclusive.

If you ascribe to the theory that health is a function of chemical balance, and too much of anything is too much for you, whether it's iron or oxygen, then you probably anticipated these results. There is a fundamental difference between administering just enough oxygen and way too much oxygen, yet the results of disparate experiments on the effects of supplemental oxygen on radiation have been lumped together, and the conclusive conclusion is that the data is inconclusive.

Scientists are quite divided on hypoxia and how to beat it. Some argue for supplemental oxygen, some against, and these scientific camps are even more split on whether or not the intake of antioxidants should be limited during radiation.

The argument against antioxidants is that they neutralize some of the free radicals produced by ionizing radiation, thus decreasing the stopping power of the applied radiation, thus making it less likely the main tumor will be killed. That's the advice I got, but only partly followed, because even then it didn't make sense.

First off, your cells can't function normally without antioxidants. It just doesn't follow they would be bad for you. Along the same lines, you can't get radiation and chemotherapy forever. Thank God. In the end, it is your body that has to fight back, and the evidence is powerful that there's no better time to supply your cells with all the tools they need to start fighting back than right now, especially if you're getting radiation.

High levels of HIF-1 make cancer cells more difficult to kill, and high levels of free radicals produced during radiation stabilize high levels of HIF-1. Antioxidants that lower levels of free radicals can lower levels of HIF-1, thus making the cancer cell more likely to die by radiation; at the same time, antioxidants are good for healthy cells.

It seems eminently reasonable to me that there might be substances out there that render cancer cells more susceptible to death by radiation, while leaving normal cells less susceptible to DNA damage. According to Warburg the difference between mutant and normal cells is that distinct, so it was with great interest that I came across a 2002 paper titled "D-alpha-Tocopheryl Succinate Enhances

Radiation-Induced Chromosomal Damage Levels in Human Cancer Cells, but Reduces it in Normal Cells."

"What," I wondered, "is D-alpha-tocopheryl succinate?"

And where could I get some?

In the produce department, as it turns out—in leafy green vegetables, whole grains, and unrefined vegetable oils. The mystery chemical was none other than vitamin E, a ranking member of the SWAT team charged with patrolling the lipid membrane for free radicals. Vitamin E has a special role because it is fat-soluble and works directly in the lipid membrane, guarding the dangling electrons on highly unsaturated fatty acids, and since vitamin E acts as a personal body guard for these vulnerable molecules, you can see why it might be a big help to add more bodyguards.

The experiment mentioned above measured the effects of radiation, vitamin E, and vitamin E plus radiation on three lines of cancer cells and three lines of normal cells. Vitamin E alone significantly increased DNA damage in cancer cells but not in normal cells, vitamin E in combination with radiation *increased* DNA damage in cancer cells in contrast to radiation alone by about a third, and vitamin E combined with radiation in normal cells *decreased* DNA damage by about a third.

It is in such data I find magic.

Vitamin E knows.

The difference between positive and negative—between increased damage on one hand and decreased damage on the other—is huge. That any single antioxidant could induce such profoundly different impacts speaks again to the fundamental nature of hypoxia in the treatment of cancer, and the evidence extends past vitamin E.

High doses of supplemental vitamin C preferentially radio-sensitized tumors in mice while providing some protection for normal cells. 10,000 IU of vitamin A taken daily for ninety days significantly reduced rectal symptoms six months after pelvic radiotherapy. Selenium, a non-metallic element that chemically resembles sulfur, is a highly efficient scavenger of free radicals, and helped improve immune response when given both during and following radiation treatment. Melatonin, the chief hormone secreted by the pineal gland, has been shown to help protect normal cells from radiation damage, and to inhibit the growth of melanoma and breast cancer cells.

It isn't just one thing, it's everything.

As a further example consider that work-horse of traditional Chinese herbal medicine, ginseng, which studies have shown is effective in combating stress, hepatitis, diabetes, and tumor growth. Nearly two hundred chemical compounds have been isolated in ginseng, including over sixty potentially active ingredients, powerful antioxidants that have been shown to both protect healthy cells and stimulate the immune response during radiation.

Spirals within spirals, waves within waves. Ginseng as medicine restores the yin of Mother Earth to an overly yang disorder, but when it comes to illustrating the inherent balances that lead to good health, even a root as Eastern as ginseng has nothing on a product as Western as whey.

Whey, a watery white liquid rich in, among other nutrients, essential amino acids, is what's left over when you make cheese. If you have a prostate or love someone who does you no doubt remember the number one indicator of high grade prostate cancer risk is high consumption of dairy products, and I'm reminded of a story.

In Montana, if you hunt ducks, and you're inexperienced, you might shoot a fish-eating duck called a Merganser. A Merganser has a strong oily taste, which requires specific cooking techniques. The traditional recipe calls for a brick to be placed in the oven along with the duck, then both duck and brick are baked for an hour at 350 degrees, at which time you throw away the duck and eat the brick.

It's the same with cheese if you're fighting prostate problems. Make up a big bunch of cheese, and then throw away the cheese. Drink the whey that's left that nature intended to balance the cheese, especially if you're getting radiation. The best radio-enhancing drugs both help kill cancer cells and actively promote the health of regular cells, and dietary supplements of whey seem to exhibit just such an effect.

The amino acids in whey are precursors to an antioxidant your cells make called *glutathione,* and when cultures are supplied with these amino acids glutathione levels tend to fall in cancer cells and rise in healthy cells. It's another case where the chemical swings both ways. The healthy cells produce more antioxidant and sustain less DNA damage, the cancer cells produce less antioxidant and sustain more DNA damage.

The idea of attacking the anaerobic nature of cancer appeals to me because you do good things for yourself instead of bad. To me, the question isn't whether lifestyle choices that lead to the proper flow and disposition of electrons can improve the effectiveness of radiation and chemotherapy; the question is whether restoring the proper flow of electrons is by itself enough to cure cancer.

If so, I'm not here to prove it.

When I needed this information most I didn't have it. When I was undergoing radiation treatment what I knew about diet and oxygen was that I might live to eat for another summer or two, or I might not. That's what I knew. There was wine in my belly, bar-b-que on my breath, and chocolate on my lips.

Ah, chocolate.

There's a Tumor in My Sweet Tooth

Sugars are carbohydrates, and a carbohydrate is exactly what it says, carbon hydrated with water. These molecules always contain twice as many hydrogen atoms as oxygen atoms, the same ratio as water, which are bonded to some number of carbon atoms, which are generally linked in rings.

The hydrating of carbon requires energy, which is generally derived from the sun. Plants make carbohydrates during photosynthesis; sunlight, carbon dioxide, and water are run through the enzymatic mixer and emerge as carbohydrates plus oxygen. Photosynthesis is the chemical opposite of respiration and the one begets the other; oxygen and carbon dioxide are mutually created and destroyed through the medium of water as plants and animals live, breathe, and swap carbohydrates.

So how can sugar be bad for you?

A particularly common carbohydrate is created when the energy in sunlight is used to combine six molecules of carbon dioxide with six molecules of water, producing one energy-rich molecule of fructose and six double-oxygen molecules. The oxygen is off-gassed into the atmosphere so you'll have something to breathe, fructose is stored as energy reserves in energy storage organs such as apples and oranges.

Fructose, the primary sugar in fruit, is built around a ring of five carbon atoms. Glucose, the sugar that fuels human cells, has the same molecular formula as fructose, but is based on a ring of six carbon atoms rather than five. Either way, glucose and fructose are simple sugars, and provide quick energy by virtue of molecular arrangements that each feature a dangling electron-rich reactive group.

It's simple to get at the energy in simple sugars, but that was too simple for scientists, who like to talk Greek, so simple sugars are also called saccharides, from the Greek for sugar. The carbon rings of simple sugars are the basic building blocks of the all the more complex carbohydrates that fill our planet; two simple sugars together are called disaccharides, while many bonded simple sugars are polysaccharides.

A common disaccharide is sucrose, everyday white table sugar, which consists of one molecule of fructose bonded to one molecule of glucose, a covalent whole that no longer dangles exposed electrons. This particular arrangement of atoms is relatively unreactive with other compounds in solutions such as your grandmother's jelly, which is why sucrose has been long used as a preservative.

Two simple sugars can join in a condensation reaction where one molecule of water is released or "condensed" during the bonding process. This bonding can take the form of either a cis bond or a trans bond. Again, this is enough to change the shape of the overall molecule and, with sugars in general, the trans bond, such as you find in sucrose, is the easier of the two for human enzymes to digest.

This matters to mammals because a third simple sugar, galactose, is produced in breasts and rarely flies solo. Instead, one molecule of galactose forms a cis bond with one molecule of glucose. This creates the disaccharide lactose, the primary sugar in breast milk, be it from people, cows, or cats. You need the enzyme lactase to digest the cis bond in lactose; if you're lactose intolerant it's because you don't have enough lactase.

Simple sugars, when they hit the human system, have immediate effect. Ten thousand years ago that didn't matter. Simple sugars were hard to come by. Fruit, honey, sugar cane, sweet potatoes—simple sugars were localized, seasonal, and diffuse. Every time you turned around you saw mastodons, not another rack of candy bars.

Your cells run on glucose, and a healthy average adult human circulates about five liters of blood that contains a total of about four to five grams of glucose. Glucose levels normally fluctuate up and down by a gram or two depending on factors such as exercise and when you last ate, but when you consistently maintain ten grams of glucose in your blood you are said to be diabetic.

Now consider that there are typically twenty to thirty grams of simple sugar in an average candy bar. It's a whopping shot of sugar, and too much glucose is toxic. When blood glucose levels rise, the hypothalamus talks to the pituitary, which tells the pancreas to produce more insulin, and by God, be quick about it.

Insulin acts on receptors all over the body to quickly reduce blood glucose levels by inducing cells to either use the glucose immediately, or to store it as a branched chain complex carbohydrate called glycogen. Problems arise because a flood of simple sugars is a metabolic emergency so dire the body tends to overreact. Too much insulin is released, which causes too much glucose to be used or stored. You get a little bit fatter, and since your insulin overreacted, you now have too little sugar in your blood, which causes the hypothalamus to call the pituitary to signal the pancreas to release glucagon.

Glucagon, a single chain peptide twenty-nine amino acids long, is the yin to insulin's yang. Throughout the body, as dynamics change, whatever you turn off, you have to turn on, and glucagon sends the message to raise glucose levels. You feel hungry, even though you just ate, and the vending machine is right down the hall.

Another candy bar completes a vicious circle.

Blood glucose levels spike.

Your body has to use that glucose somehow, and fermentation requires nineteen times as much glucose to provide the same amount of energy as respiration. A flood of glucose is like a chemical mandate to ferment, and fermentation is basic to the nature of cancer. In hypoxic cancer cells primed with HIF-1 to extract energy from fermentation as necessary, that shot of glucose would go down like manna from heaven.

It's exactly what the doctor didn't order.

So, why are our radiation waiting rooms stocked with cookies?

How can a manufacturer claim a cereal is healthy because a serving contains one gram of fiber when it also contains fifteen grams of sugar? How can anyone claim their product is better for you after simply swapping one simple sugar for another? At first glance, it doesn't make sense, until you look at it in terms of those plays where someone sits around looking at a chair while waiting for someone who isn't going to show up.

It's the Theater of the Absurd and, if you have tickets you don't want, consider how likely it is that cancer responds to fluctuating glucose levels the same way it reacts to cycling oxygen levels, by evolving. Cancer cells can take advantage of high glucose levels whereas healthy cells can't. Not only that, after months or years of spirited combat against wildly fluctuating blood glucose levels, our bodies tend to give up the fight, which is where diabetes rears its sickly head.

If you want to blame something, blame the Pleistocene. Simple sugars simply weren't available in the everyday diet of the humans who gave us the genes that give us our enzymes. Our enzymes are adapted instead to the sugars that were more generally available over the past millions instead of past dozens of years, complex carbohydrates.

Complex carbohydrates are polysaccharides, or chains of simple sugars longer than two, and generally much longer. It takes extra reactions to get at the energy stored in the simple sugars and, by controlling the rate of these reactions, the glucose can be released slowly over time as your cells ask for it.

Glycogen, a branched chain of glucose molecules our cells use to store energy, is a complex carbohydrate. Starch, a long and relatively unbranched chain of glucose molecules, is another. Plants like potatoes store energy as starch because unbranched chains save on storage space and, when linear chains of starch bond to their neighbors, you have another complex carbohydrate, cellulose.

The glucose molecules in cellulose share electrons in three dimensions, forming a bonded lattice that is not broken down by human enzymes. Cows and termites have the chemicals to digest cellulose, but people don't, and undigested cellulose is the dietary fiber that exercises the digestive track while scouring it of potentially cancerous polyps.

I fish in cow country so I know cow pies. A pie fresh from the cow is about as disgusting as anything in the pantheon of nature. It's formless stinking slime. All the fiber is gone, and if you don't get enough fiber, that cow pie is the state of your gut. There's nothing for your bowels to work with, nothing to push. The mush stays put, and in that stagnant mush of low dietary fiber are many links to many diseases, all of which should come as no surprise to anyone who's ever had the misfortune of meeting up with the north end of a south bound cow.

So why would you ever want to go on a low carbohydrate diet?

Plants use the power of the sun to build cellulose and starch, and they also use the power of the sun to build molecules that protect that cellulose and starch. Bound up in all that complex carbohydrate are all manner of vitamins and antioxidants and other specialized chemicals that plant needs to survive. Different plants have evolved different systems of coordinated chemical defense, and what works for a rutabaga works for you.

Plant and animal cells face similar challenges in managing oxygen, and pollen from medicinal plants has been found in 60,000-year-old Neanderthal burial sites. People have been using medicinal plants for as long as anybody can remember because they work, and recent research describes hundreds of chemicals in dozens of plants that alter in all kinds of ways the Pony Express system of chemical messengers that is you.

As examples of interest to cancer patients, the various active ingredients in substances as diverse as green tea, fish oil, selenium, and curcumin (found in the spice turmeric) have all been shown to inhibit angiogenesis in tumors. Silymarin, the active ingredient in milk thistle, seems to interrupt cancer cell division, to keep cancer cells from spreading, to shorten the time cancer cells live, and to inhibit tumor angiogenesis, in part by acting at sex hormone receptors to severely restrict growth factor proteins.

The idea that plants stimulate human sex receptors is, on the face of it, pretty darn kinky. A little quality time with the family sheep pales in comparison to getting it on with the azaleas. This isn't interspecies sex, it's interkingdom sex, and what it really gets at is how, as cellular beings on the planet Earth, we're all in this together.

Some plants are such concentrated bundles of human goodness it's like they're designed by a higher power, and no cancer book would be complete without discussing the Brassica family of plants. This is the family of cruciferous vegetables, including kale, cabbage, rutabagas, cauliflower, Brussels sprouts, bok choy, and, of course, broccoli.

Mustard, horseradish, and wasabi are also Brassicas, and the distinctive tang of these foods is a manifestation of the chemical defenses this family evolved over the eons against grazing animals. Brassica plants contain an enzyme that when mixed with animal saliva creates a small organic molecule that tastes hot in the mouth.

The molecule created by chewing is so reactive plants can't store it directly, and it bothered chewing ruminants of the world enough they turned to other food sources. On the other hand it's quite tasty when mixed with ginger and served over sushi, and a 2003 study found that the presence of this tiny molecule also led to significantly increased apoptosis in several prostate cancer cell lines, with minimal effects on normal cells.

Broccoli contains this molecule, along with high concentrations of another short nitrogen- and sulfur-containing molecule, sulforaphane. This particular molecule inhibits production of a Phase I enzyme that activates potential carcinogens, and stimulates production of a Phase II enzyme that destroys carcinogens. So, chemicals in broccoli destroy potential carcinogens, de-activate carcinogens that make it through, and help cells that have gone over to the dark side do the decent thing and kill themselves.

Assisted ritual cell suicide, now there's a vegetable with talents. But wait, there's more.

Broccoli isn't generally touted as one of the more sensuous vegetables but again this is a plant where interkingdom receptor intercourse rears its promiscuous head. A 2001 population based study in Sweden found eating one to two servings a day of crucifers, such as broccoli or cabbage, lowered overall breast cancer incidence by 20-40 percent, possibly by shifting the estrogen pathway. Other studies on both rodents and humans indicate that chemicals in cruciferous vegetables are bisexual, because they work on both androgen and estrogen receptors, and help both men and women in a spectrum of hormone-related cancers, including breast, cervical, prostate, and endometrial.

But cruciferous vegetables are more than just the occasional one night stand against cancer. They also reduce cellular oxidative stress, which is a prime cause of aging, at least according to a 2006 study partially funded by the National Institutes of Health.

This study compared the effects on twenty people of eating two cups of raw Brassica vegetables per day, as opposed to eating artificial multivitamin and fiber supplements substituted for the vegetables. Each diet was followed for four weeks, and urine samples were collected daily, and then analyzed for F_2-isoprostane, a fat that is produced when free radicals oxidize the most common highly unsaturated fatty acid in your cell membranes.

This fat is part of your Pony Express system of chemical messengers, and think of it as a cry for help. The more of it there is in your blood, the more your cells are crying out for antioxidants to combat free radicals. The level of this chemical messenger is used as a "bio-marker" of overall systemic oxidative stress that leads to aging and cancer, and levels dropped 22 percent during the diet of raw vegetables as compared to control, but only a negligible 0.2 percent when on a diet of multivitamin and fiber supplements.

There's no thing like the real thing.

This study focused on raw cruciferous vegetable intake because all processing, even cooking, destroys some nutrients. Comparing the effects of vitamin C on health by comparing diets rich in raw apples, processed orange juice from concentrate, and hard pills in a plastic bottle is like comparing, well, apples and oranges. It's confounding, and if you don't want to eat your vegetables, you can find plenty of science to back you up.

For instance, studies show oxidative stress was lowered by lycopene (found in tomatoes), fruit juice, and broccoli. Other studies show oxidative stress is not lowered by fruit and vegetables in general, carrot juice, spinach, processed vegetable burgers, and antioxidant supplements. So, the bad news is that processed vegetable burgers don't cure cancer, the good news is you don't have to eat them.

What are these guys thinking? Somebody must have known the congressman's brother-in-law to get that study funded. If it seems absurd that's because it is.

Which brings us back to radiation.

During my half-life as a dirty bomb I ate a couple flax oil smoothies a week. I've always eaten vegetables and whole grains, but, realistically, at that time I'd say half my daily calories came from the plant kingdom, half from animals. I still ate trans fat laden products like flour tortillas, crackers, and frozen pizzas, plus plenty of simple sugar laden foods like low fat salad dressings, and cookies at the hospital, because, as much money as I was giving them, I figured I ought to get something besides X-rays.

Bad plan.

As far as my diet during radiation, on a scale of one to ten, I give myself a four. I fed my cancer plenty of trans fats and simple sugars; my healthy cells didn't get nearly the tools they needed to countermand the most stressful oxidative situation they would ever encounter. There was plenty I could have done to better take advantage of that 80 percent variation in the response of cells to radiation, and I wish I had, because it's not like I endured all that ionizing radiation without side effects.

How come I'm always scratching my ass?

Because it always itched, and when I answered myself this question about mid-way through my radiotherapy, I wondered why it had taken me so long to realize this was no ordinary rash, but instead radiation burn. I treated it the same way I treat all burns, whether they're from the sun or the woodstove, with raw slices of juicy aloe vera from the cactus I grow in the south window of my house.

I used a fresh slice every time, rubbed it in whenever the burn itched, every couple hours for the next couple of days; by then the skin was back to normal and I could stop walking around with my hand down the back of my pants. I felt proud of my minor achievement, and the next time I saw the radiation doctor I asked him what he thought of aloe as a...

"It doesn't really work," he interrupted, and then quoted specifically and knowledgably from a study in which aloe had been shown to be no more effective than placebo at treating radiation burned skin.

"Try this," he said, then wrote me a prescription.

The conversation hadn't gone at all like I'd expected. I opened my mouth, trying to figure out how I could now say that since aloe had worked so well on my outsides, I was thinking about taking an edible form of aloe that might work similarly well on my insides, and what did he think of that...

Anticipating the wrong question, he raised both hands palm out.

"And no," he said, "I don't know what it costs."

I fulfilled my role in this act of the Theater of Absurd by thanking him for the prescription. There was no point in ruffling his feathers, but what I really wanted to tell him was that aloe worked a hell of a lot better than his X-ray machine.

I never did try that edible aloe and I wish I had. I could have eaten way more antioxidant-rich vegetables. The rectum adjoins the prostate. If I'd done everything I could to protect my healthy cells from that onslaught of radiation-induced free radicals, maybe right now I wouldn't be spending such a disconcerting number of days with a slightly bleeding butt for company, but, still, I count myself as lucky.

As it is, the fix is as quick as more frequent trips to the underwear store.

It could have been so much worse.

The power to the X-ray machine was consistently interrupted throughout the duration of my treatment, the clamor of the mechanism dying to silence in the glow of the flashing red emergency lights. Something was wrong, and if they knew what it was, you'd think they would have fixed it. There was just so much chance that mistakes could be made, and maybe they were, who knows?

That's the way my daily treatment went. I'd lie there, either getting radiation, or waiting for the power to come back on so I could get more radiation. X-Ray Lady would come and go. Sometimes we'd talk and joke like it was nothing out of the ordinary to have flashing red lights on the walls; mostly I'd lay there not moving except to breathe, pretending I was somewhere else as X-ray Lady changed the lead shields that changed the shape of the radiation entering my body.

One day near the end of my treatment we were talking and she said:

"Looks like I'll be moving on, probably next month."

"You're kidding," I said. "You got fired?"

She laughed. "No, no, no," she said, "Nothing like that. It's just that they're getting a new X-ray machine so I figured it's time for me to retire too."

A new machine wouldn't be in time for me but it would be for the next guy.

"That's great," I said. "Wow."

She changed the lead plate, then left the room and hit the switch. Around me the relic whined like a tractor with a bad clutch and clanked to a proper stop. That dose administered, X-Ray Lady came back in to prepare for the next dose.

"So," I said, "What do they do with this old machine when the new one arrives?"

"They sold this one back to a place in Boston," she said.

Few cities in the world have higher standards of medicine than Boston and it made no sense whatsoever.

"Boston?" I said. "What would a hospital back east want with this old thing?"

"Oh it's not going to a hospital," she said. "They sold it to a veterinarian."

At least that explained why they hadn't bothered to fix the machine.

"If it's good enough for Fido," I replied, "it's good enough for me."

Reefer Madness

The truth is those X-rays and that machine terrified me. Most days I wanted to cry instead of laugh. I never could have joked about my predicament if it weren't for a drug whose side effects include a desire to listen to the White Album backwards.

I hadn't smoked much pot since college and, in the age of medical marijuana, it's gotten a lot stronger. A couple hits in the parking lot and whoopee. My body may have been in that machine but the rest of me wasn't. Most days I snorkeled colorful coral reefs in my mind, as far from my drab concrete reality as I could imagine, absorbing the radiation in a state of concentration as close to rapture as I could achieve.

I hesitated to include this chapter because it's a divisive issue, but marijuana was too appropriate a topic to ignore for four reasons. First, the social and political stigma attached to marijuana use is true of all medicinal plant use, only more so. Second, well-studied hemp is a paradigm of typical differences between plants and pharmaceuticals based on those plants. Third, research into marijuana revealed a fundamental chemical link between the nervous and immune systems of animals, and, in the end, if you're going to beat cancer, it will be your immune system that does it.

And, fourth, it's too good an opportunity to make jokes to pass up.

As far as medicine goes, we tend to underestimate the importance of a good laugh. As far as social and political stigma go, the moment of original sin for me came in the early seventies. It was a couple of weeks into my freshman year of college. I was on the swim team, on the return trip from a match against another college, and we were stopped for no discernable reason at a set of railroad tracks on a back road on a dark night in the middle of Pennsylvania.

Red autumn maples crowded into the beam of the headlights from both sides, and Taz, the driver, sat there contentedly tapping his fingers to the power riffs of the first Jefferson Starship album. Me, I marveled at the notes of the first electric fiddle I'd ever heard, and wondered what we were waiting for. Kelly, the team captain, was riding shotgun, and smiling at Taz as if time would never end.

Taz withered under the knowing smile and gradually quit tapping his fingers.

"There is no train, is there?" he said.

My God, I thought, he's on drugs.

"No," replied Kelly, "There's not."

Taz took the news philosophically.

"You better drive," he said.

The ice broken, Nancy, another freshman and sitting to my right, pulled out the first bag of pot I'd ever seen and began to roll a joint. I'd been taught that this was the time to open the door and walk home, but I was going to spend the next four years swimming with these people. If I left, I'd always be the guy who left, and the truth is dope fiends were a lot more interesting than I'd been led to believe in church.

Plus, dope fiends sure seemed to know a lot of girls.

Some of them *were* girls.

And the one beside me smelled of chlorine and coconut shampoo.

Such were my thoughts as the joint went counterclockwise around the car, until finally reaching Kelly, who was now sitting in the driver's seat directly in front of me. He smoked at the joint a couple a times, then held it back over his shoulder for me to grab. I'd decided the best course under the circumstances was to fake a hit, but I was both tentative and unfamiliar with the finger-to-finger push experienced smokers employ. I fumbled the hand-off and the burning joint disappeared into the jumble of wadded fast food wrappers at my feet.

"God damn," observed Nancy, "He dropped it."

There was no faking it now. By the time I dug the joint from the skinned over ketchup and leftover french fries everybody was staring at me. Life has moments when a thing you do influences everything that happens forever after. For me, that's how one of them happened, peer pressure, plain and simple, and no sooner had I sucked on the joint than I began coughing it back up.

Nancy pounded me on the back and smiled.

"Good hit," she said.

Smoke entered my lungs, chemicals entered my blood.

Marijuana contains over sixty active ingredients called cannabinoids (kuh-NAB-i-noids) that interact with cannabinol (kuh-NAB-i-nawl) protein receptors found in some but not all cells. The discovery of these receptors was big news in the 1970's because it meant people produce their own cannabinoids to act on those receptors, chemicals that represent the ultimate in home-grown, and the first such molecule to be isolated was called anandamide (a-NAN-duh-mide) after the Sanskrit word for bliss.

Now there's a scientist with a flair for words.

Cannabinol receptors appear in mammals as early as the first cell division of a fertilized egg. They're found in an evolutionarily diverse array of animals, including leeches, mollusks, chickens, turtles, trout, fruit flies, and even, in about as primitive of an animal as exists, the microscopic hydra.

Hydra are thought to date back 800 million years or so to the beginnings of animal life, and are built like jellyfish, only smaller. A simple fresh-water hydra is a flexible elongated tube of jelly from which tentacles extend. The jelly filled tube contains primitive internal organs; the tentacles contain poison-tipped harpoons loaded into membrane-contained firing chambers.

Now imagine a bacteria cell whipping a thin tail as it swims up against a hydra tentacle, bending hairs that cause calcium ions to stream from the affected firing chamber. There are those electrons again. The gush of moving ions out of the firing chamber triggers a return gush of water into the firing chamber, which in turn inflates and extends a coiled hollow tube capped with a poisoned harpoon.

From hair to harpoon it's one of the fastest reactions in biology and takes only nanoseconds. The process is coordinated by a simple nervous system, among the first in the kingdom of animals, and right from the get-go the nervous system that controlled this predatory response needed an off-switch.

Poisoned barbed harpoons are a ruthlessly efficient way of gathering food. You can see where the first couple of hydra might have eaten until they exploded. Animals eat, early animals needed to stop eating before they'd eaten too much, and a 1999 study showed anandamide activity at cannabinoid receptors in hydra provided just such a retrograde reaction to inhibit the feeding response.

Cannabinoids work upstream to stop the effect before it comes. Instead of building a bigger dam, cannabinoids make it stop raining. It's a handy trick, and once this retrograde switch was genetically engineered, cells, as they so often do, continued to use the chemical innovation in other applications. These chemicals are fundamental to the primary processes of animal life, including seeing, eating, reproducing, defending, and thinking; yet, of all the plants on this green Earth, only hemp synthesizes significant concentrations of cannabinoids.

What's up with that?

Some say it's God's plan, others chalk it up to evolutionary coincidence, still others invoke the Devil. Many plants are spread by making themselves appealing to animal species; perhaps marijuana has qualities that make it useful to humans for that very reason. If so, it picked the right species to befriend.

Hemp fibers have been found in Asian archaeological digs dating back to about 10,000 years ago. Early uses of hemp included clothes and rope, and the technological innovation of rope led to sailing ships that crossed the oceans. Hemp was cultivated all over the world as a cash crop, and as recently as 1942 the patriotic infomercial "Hemp for Victory" exhorted Americans to grow hemp to support the World War II effort.

The development of synthetic nylon slashed the market for hemp rope, but, like any successful multi-national corporation, hemp is diversified in its portfolio of human appeal. In the face of decreased demand for fiber, hemp turned to pharmaceuticals, with the result that few modern plants are as widely spread or as pampered.

The first recorded medical use of hemp was nearly 5,000 years ago. At the time the pyramids were a fairly new feature in Egypt, while in China Emperor Shen Neng prescribed cannabis tea for gout, malaria, beriberi, and rheumatism. The emperor also researched natural ephedra, the raw ingredient in methamphetamine, and if he ever self-tested the combined effects of both drugs, it may explain why legend had it he could look into his own belly to observe the effects of the plants he ate.

Medicinal use of marijuana spread westward over the coming millennia, and generations of doctors prescribed hemp for ailments as diverse as epilepsy, nausea, menstrual cramps, multiple sclerosis, and sleep and vision problems. That's a lot to ask of one plant, yet there is a pharmacological basis for all these treatments and more.

For example, cannabinoid receptors are prevalent in eye parts that maintain fluid pressure. Too much intraocular fluid pressure pinches the optic nerve at the back of the eyeball, which causes glaucoma, and many corroborating studies show marijuana use lowers intraocular eye pressure and helps alleviate glaucoma.

Other historically touted benefits of marijuana seem at first glance to be more fancy than fact. Consider the year 1597, when the Briton John Gerard, in his popular book on medicinal plants, recommended hemp "as it consumeth wind and drieth up seed," the seed in this case being semen and the wind anal in nature.

Modern medicine has yet to show marijuana cures common flatulence, yet animal and human research has shown cannabinoids reduce sperm count and motility. In one experiment men who smoked eight joints a day for a month produced fewer sperm that were less active. The study also found the effects were reversible, and after eight joints a day for a month there is no record on whether the men had any trouble finding their penises.

H-m-m, maybe I left it with the car keys.

If you're a mammal you had to learn to suckle at mama's breast, and high levels of cannabinoids concentrated on the day of birth in brains cells associated with feeding behavior stimulate receptors that trigger this feeding response. The levels of triggering brain chemicals drop drastically on the second day of life, and the urge to suckle would disappear if it were not for another supply of cannabinoids available to the infant, and that supply is in the mother's milk. It appears that a newborn brain produces high levels of cannabinoids just long enough to initiate the feeding response, at which point similar molecules in the mother's milk provide the chemical reinforcement to continue.

Suckling is one of the first skills we learn, and, I hope, one of the last we forget. Guys seem obsessed with breasts because they are. Of course, so are women, or saline and silicone wouldn't be such big business. The chemistry runs deep, and it should come as no surprise that cannabinoids effectively treat eating disorders, for what are the "munchies" if not the suckling response revisited in adult form?

Vomiting and nausea are significant side effects of chemotherapy. Some people become so conditioned to the coming cytotoxins they throw up at the mere sight of the hospital. An inability to keep down food significantly limits overall survival rates; antiemetics are drugs that reduce these symptoms, and a 1975 experiment published in the prestigious *New England Journal of Medicine* examined the potential of marijuana to reduce vomiting and nausea.

Twenty chemotherapy patients who had not responded to traditional antiemetic drugs were given either placebo or cannabinoids two hours prior to treatment; results showed these hard-to-treat patients experienced significant relief from cannabinoids as opposed to placebo with minimal side effects. Subsequent experiments substantiated the therapeutic effects of cannabinoids on vomiting and nausea, while other studies showed a positive effect on appetite.

Anorexia and weight loss are common side effects of both cancer and cancer treatments, affecting perhaps half of newly diagnosed patients. The food you don't eat can't help you, and as little as a 5 percent loss in body weight has been associated with reduced survival rates. Cannabinoids are effective at treating nutritional disorders because they come at the problem from both angles; they help you to eat more, and they help you keep down what you do manage to eat.

After early studies showed marijuana reduced nausea and increased appetite in chemotherapy patients, industry took a time-honored tack when it comes to medicinal plants in general, which was to develop a profit-generating pharmaceutical that could be prescribed in lieu of the non-profit-generating plant; year-long clinical trials on the effects of the first such chemical were begun on both monkeys and dogs.

The dog trial was abandoned when animals began dying of convulsions, while monkeys showed no observable significantly adverse effects. This led to the conclusion the drug was safe to test on people, and during clinical trials on humans "virtually all the patients who received this drug experienced at least one adverse reaction." This led to the conclusion the drug was ready to be marketed, despite widespread adverse reactions of the central nervous system, including vertigo, ataxia (unsteady movements due to inability to regulate posture), dysphoria (anxiety, depression, or unease), and depersonalization (no explanation needed).

This particular chemical is generally described as a synthetic version of naturally occurring tetra-hydro-cannabinol (THC), but it's not. The molecules differ in the location of reactive double bonds; they differ in the number of atoms they contain. These very different molecules are metabolized in very different ways, and the differences between the medical properties of the whole plant and the synthetic drug don't stop there.

There are over four hundred chemicals in a marijuana plant, including sixty-six different cannabinoids. Any or all of these chemicals could contribute to the overall effect of the plant as medicine. Nobody knows for sure, yet a great deal of research shows complex interactions between the active ingredients tend to limit negative side effects. This is in part because the chemicals together buffer the rate and fashion in which they are metabolized, and various ratios of active ingredients affect receptors in various ways.

Medical marijuana growers have reputedly capitalized on this knowledge by breeding various strains that contain different proportions of active ingredients, and therefore have different therapeutic effects on the human body. Some strains are said to tend to make people hungry, some to induce sleep, some to reduce anxiety, and some to, well, as the scientists put it, increase euphoria.

Call me crazy, but I'll take euphoria over depersonalization any day.

There are an estimated 300 million pot smokers worldwide. Statistically, it's a huge sample, and the disorders of the central nervous system associated with the imitation THC simply aren't associated with the plant as a whole. In terms of addiction, a 1990 study ranked marijuana as fourteenth out of eighteen commonly consumed drugs, behind number one nicotine, number eight alcohol, and number twelve caffeine.

This is a drug that's easier than most to kick when it's time, but the point isn't that you should smoke pot. The point is that this is a well studied plant with well studied pharmaceutical analogues. Marijuana offers insight into the differences between the effects of plants and pills in general, because the entire mélange of natural chemicals in a whole plant has a much different effect on the human body than does a molecular imposter of any single constituent chemical.

It didn't surprise me that four billion years of cellular evolution could provide a mix of molecules that my own cells could more easily tolerate, but I was very surprised that cannabinoids have been shown to shrink tumors and destroy cancer cells. Research dating back to 1975, both in vitro and in vivo, on nine cancers, including prostate, breast, lung, thyroid, and skin, has demonstrated at least four chemical pathways by which cannabinoids may exert anticancer cellular effect. These reactions tend to spare normal cells while inducing apoptosis in cancer cells, and at the same time inhibiting the growth, angiogenesis, and metastasis of tumors.

Now there's a non-confrontational approach to tumor control. "Hey...you...the mutant...I got this especially for you."

Experiencing euphoria, the cancer cell then sees the light.

"Oh...wow...I had no idea...please allow me to kill myself."

Researchers are split on the effectiveness of medicinal plants. Still, overall, the research indicates that the medicinal effects of plants tend to be muted—for both the good and the bad—as compared to pills. In other words, the chemical mix in any given plant may not be enough to impart immediate and overwhelming relief, but it's also less likely to cause harm when taken over time.

This is not to say all plants are good, or all potent pharmaceuticals are bad. They're just different. Sometimes you need that chemical kick in the pants. For instance, radioactivity inflamed my prostate, which choked down my urethra, the main exit tube for urine. This results in what TV calls "a going problem," and before my radioactive seed implantation procedure, the nurse advised me that a widely advertised drug was routinely prescribed and would be part of my regimen.

"Sure," I said. "How long will I have to take it?"

"Many men will take it for the rest of their lives," she replied.

"What?" I said.

It's just another one of those things you learn along the way.

I was determined I wouldn't be one of those statistics who used that urinary aid drug for the rest of their life. It just seemed like one step closer to a diaper. On the other hand, during my radioactive peak, I couldn't pee without it. Even so, I tried. I took the smallest effective dose, about a third of what the manufacturer recommended. I cut back on diuretics like coffee, I drank lots of water. Within six weeks I was off the stuff for good, which completely alleviated another adverse effect.

That being the number of dollars in my wallet.

These drugs are expensive for everybody. They're expensive to buy, they're expensive to produce, and they're especially expensive to research. Because of the costs involved, most pharmaceuticals are tested on a few dozen to a few hundred people for a couple of weeks or months. We simply don't know the long term effects of these drugs, while some medicinal plants have been tested on hundreds of millions of people for thousands of years. This evidence is disregarded as non-double-blind nonsense, yet, again, well studied marijuana is an example of a plant in which modern double-blind data corroborates historical population-based inferences.

In terms of numbers, a 1999 study showed 76 million Americans admitted to smoking dope, including 9 percent of the population in the last year, and 5 percent in the last month. Five percent of 300 million Americans is...let's see now...this is the kind of thing you might worry about if you smoke a lot of pot because it has been shown to affect math skills...that's fifteen million people wondering how it might affect memory.

There is plenty of evidence it does, particularly in the short term.

Some degree of forgetfulness is the price you pay for euphoria.

Now what were we talking about again?

Hippocampus is Greek for *seahorse*, and the hippocampus is a seahorse-shaped organ buried deep in the primitive brain. Perceptions—sights, sounds, smells—come in the tail end of the seahorse, pass through five neurally distinct regions, and emerge at the head end as (ten to fifteen second) short term memories ready to be either stored or forgotten. If the hippocampus isn't the seat of consciousness it's at least a footstool, and this memory organ is particularly rich in cannabinoid receptors.

As you would expect, stimulating these receptors with marijuana affects the formation of short term memories. In a 1971 study, 150 college students who had used the drug at least twelve times were asked 200 questions about what they thought it was like to be high on marijuana. As far as short term memory during intoxication goes, 65 percent of the subjects admitted to forgetting the beginning of a sentence by the time they got to the end; there is no record of how long those sentences were.

A girl I knew in college could go on for days.

Now what was her name again?

The effect of chronic marijuana use on long term memory has also been the subject of scrutiny. One 1973 study tested thirty using and twenty-four non-using Jamaican men on fifteen cognitive tests, and found no significant differences in the mental performance of long term users and non-users. Marijuana users in this test were sober (or said they were) at the time of the test, but had smoked an average of twenty joints a day for the past ten years; no extra credit was given for remembering to show up at all.

On the other hand an Indian study examined the effects of marijuana on mental processes in twenty-five smokers, twenty-five bhang (a cannabis beverage) drinkers, and twenty-five controls. Statistical differences were found in eight of ten cognitive tests, including time perception, memory, size estimation, motor speed, and reaction time. Most differences were minor; in a memory test involving remembering words from a list the difference averaged about a word. Some differences were greater; word association reaction time nearly doubled in smokers compared to non-smokers, but that could have been because subjects were trying to think of words that weren't just correct but meaningful.

The effect of marijuana on memory is no laughing matter. Of course, it's no crying matter either. Complex tasks seem to be affected more than simple tasks, but studies involving casual users seldom find cognitive differences and, even with heavy long term use, changes in cognitive abilities tend to be subtle rather than extreme.

For instance, in one study group heavy long term use was defined as about an ounce a month for twenty-four years, while short term heavy use in a second group was about an ounce a month for ten years. Each group was compared to a control group on nine cognitive tests; the people who smoked heavily for ten years did slightly better on most tests than the control group, the group that smoked heavily for twenty-four years did slightly worse, and the greatest disparity between smokers and non-smokers was in the ability to estimate the passage of time without counting off the seconds.

So why is this plant so vilified?

It is medicine of a fundamental order, it's so inexpensive you can grow it yourself, and it's relatively non-addictive. Despite media hype to the contrary, side effects are generally minimal, and include euphoria as opposed to depersonalization, yet even though marijuana is legal as medicine in Montana, it's tough to find a doctor who will discuss it, much less prescribe it.

In this, marijuana is just a well publicized example of the institutional and educational bias against medicinal plants in general. At the same time, there are plants out there that would just as soon kill you as have you look at them. Whether with plants or pills you mess with your Pony Express system of chemical messengers at your own peril, which is why it's worth getting a second opinion.

If you are truly interested in doing everything you can to get rid of cancer don't just talk to oncologists. Talk to dieticians, talk to naturopaths. Natural doctors are just like regular doctors, there are good ones and bad ones. Find someone you can talk to, get the rest of the story, then make up your own mind.

This is particularly true if you've just gone through conventional cancer treatment. Your cells have just taken one of the worst beatings they're ever going to get. They need all the help you can give them—both for themselves, and because it is very unlikely that every last cancer cell in your body has been destroyed. This is the point at which your cells have to take over the fight, and, from broccoli to flax, there's lots of evidence that lots of plants can help root out the invaders.

The point of most plant-based medicines is to make you healthy in a week or a month, and keep you that way. It's more of a slow shift back into balance, as opposed to a quick pharmaceutical fix, which we sometimes need, but which leads to between 1.3 million and 15 million adverse drug reactions in America each year. The chances of adverse effects, including death, rise greatly as you combine drugs, and our culture of poly-pharmacy is a far cry from the Hippocratic doctrines that instruct physicians to at least do no harm.

Medical advice is dispensed based on what we know today, which is not what we'll know tomorrow. Drugs interfere with chemicals that haven't even been discovered yet, and there is no telling what other crucially important bodily interactions remain hidden simply because it's so difficult to find that which you don't seek.

In this, medicine is no different than life.

Finding a needle in a haystack is child's play compared to isolating a protein in the hundred trillion cells that make up a human body, and this is particularly true if you don't know the protein is there. Scientists went looking for cannabinoid receptors only after it was determined that marijuana wasn't reacting with any of the known receptors at the time. What they found, after years of searching, was a protein that was far more important to the animal kingdom of cells than anybody would have ever guessed.

Just as early animals would have had to control the feeding response, so would they have battled pathogens. Eating and defending would be among the first tasks emerging nervous systems managed as a whole, and cannabinoid receptors are concentrated in both nervous and immune cells. Intriguingly, immune receptors are a distinctly different protein than receptors in the nervous system, although they respond to the same chemicals, which implies evolution to or from the same place in response to a common need, and one common need was certainly communication.

The emerging brain would have had to communicate with the emerging immune system, to exchange signals and issue instructions, and in the final analysis, whether you're battling swine flu or old age or cancer, your immune system must carry the day. Despite several demonstrated chemical pathways between brain and immune cells, including cannabinoid receptors, most experts belittle the idea that you can consciously improve the quality of your immune system.

Should you believe them?

The Kiss of Death

The cells that are you fight a battle against pathogens that begins with conception and continues until your final breath. Cancer is just one of the foes hoping to establish residence in that delightfully warm, nutritious blood you circulate. Your immune system is on the front lines of this perpetual battle with the forces of darkness, and one of your first layers of defense is the molecular equivalent of Sicilian-style bag men.

These bag men are comprised of over twenty proteins called the *complement* system, which circulate constantly in your blood. These proteins go from cell to cell, banging on doors at all hours of the day and night, demanding proof that you are you, proof that each cell must present in the form of molecular identification fragments.

When your cells build fats and proteins they also build fragments that identify you as you, and those identifying chemical segments are presented to the outside world as offerings on protein altars extruding from the plasma cell membrane. These intricate protein altars, the major histocompatability complex (MHC), are a veritable dance of intertwined peptide chains that span the cell membrane and end on the outside in a folded clump. This folded clump has a central groove that holds the molecular identifiers like a bun holds a hot dog, and it is on this Oscar-Mayer of an altar that the offerings are made that prove that you are you.

Make the right offering, and the complement proteins move on. But suppose a cell misses an offering, or even worse, makes the wrong offering. This can happen when a virus takes over the genetic production of one of your cells. The chemicals being manufactured are no longer your chemicals, they are the virus's chemicals. Molecular evidence of this invasion is presented on the cell membrane, and the bag men move in.

The bag men can break a few cellular knees; they can even kill cells outright by causing membranes to rupture. The problem with outright rupture is that whatever was in the affected cell is released into the bloodstream, which can be counterproductive, particularly with viral DNA. So, rather than bursting (or lysing) the cell, the complement proteins attach to the membrane of the offending cell, thus marking it for death.

It's like waking up with a big X spray-painted on your door. The hit men are coming, and among the first responders to the appearance of an intruder are natural killers. These cells were discovered and named in the 1970's because it was thought they killed naturally, i.e., without provocation, but this has since been shown to be a false premise.

Natural killers do need a stimulus to act, but the transcendent beauty of this cell is that its receptors react to many stimuli, not just one. Natural killers are designed to evaluate what is you and what isn't you. If they're not sentient, they're close to it. They can act if a cell presents the wrong identification but, unlike many other immune cells, they can also act if a cell doesn't present enough of the right identification.

Natural killers make decisions and act upon them, and are part of an *innate immune system* that has features in common with animals as diverse as insects and mollusks. Each and every creature has its own unique molecular identity, and I don't know if this means that clams and mosquitoes have a sense of self, but it does mean the alphabet soup of chemicals that natural killers sample in humans is complex.

At least a couple dozen mutually interacting molecules are likely to be involved in the decision as to friend or foe. Some offerings on the protein altars tip the scales toward death, some offerings toward life, and some offerings carry more weight than others. An alien bacteria cell painted with complement proteins is marked for certain death, but all the decisions aren't so easy.

This is particularly true of cancer cells, since they once came from you, and are therefore more likely to offer up acceptable parts of you. It is identity theft, pure and simple, but any mutant's papers aren't perfect, and natural killers are among the most adept of your immune cells at sniffing out inconsistencies. Natural killers act as judge, jury, and executioner on the sum of evidence both pro and con, are generally regarded as one of the body's most important defenses against cancer, and administer swift justice.

Natural killers attack by first attaching themselves to the offending cell, and then releasing chemicals so deadly they must be stored in protective granules. The first chemical, perforin, perforates the cell membrane of the imposter, which allows a second round of chemicals called granzymes to enter into the alien cell and induce apoptosis.

Apoptosis is programmed cell death occurring in ritualistic fashion with an eye toward recycling. DNA fragments, the cell membrane collapses in on itself. The end result is that the larger cell dissolves into a bunch of smaller membrane-contained bubbles, and all the original cytoplasm in the dying cell is contained in those new bubbles. Nothing escapes, and the bubbles and their contents are now ready to be either recycled or destroyed.

You're quite good at dismantling cells into reusable parts without spilling. You do it billions of times every day, in response to many factors, including low levels of oxygen or high levels of free radicals. These cells are doing nothing more than the right thing for the common good and, following apoptosis, the neatly packaged cell fragments are quickly disposed of by another type of immune cell called *macrophages.*

Macrophages clean up after hit men but also attack on their own. They're large cells, marvels of bioengineering designed to reach out and envelop either waste or prey in an oversized flexible membrane hanging like a shroud from a central manufacturing sphere. The shroud membrane contains granules of digestive juices that begin working on contact. Digestion is swift, and proof of death is required. Hit men might present the capo with a finger, but macrophages display antigens.

Antigens is simply the name scientists have given to the identifying chemicals of the intruding life form. Macrophages isolate and save the antigens, and then present them on MHC protein altars of their own, where the information is noted by the middle men in the *acquired immune system,* helper T cells.

Innate immune cells like natural killers respond quickly at the source but lack numbers to neutralize major infections. Your acquired immune system takes longer to mobilize but responds in force, like the main army arriving to relieve advance troops. Assembling this army requires both time and energy, and is dependent on a high level of communication between several different types of highly specialized immune cells.

These cells all hang out together in your spleen, and when presented with antigens react in a couple of important ways. First, they create antibodies in response to those antigens, and second, they issue instructions that result in the cloning of a large army of what we'll call killer T cells that are also specific to that antigen.

The antigen identifies and is produced by the invader, the antibody is a chemical you produce that identifies and reacts with the antigen. Antibodies, once built, attach to the antigens on the invading cell, and it's like another great big X on the door.

Antibodies can interfere with the function of the targeted cell, and they signal in killer T cells, natural killers, macrophages, and the rest of the immune army. Not only that, but the genetic code for that particular antigen is stored away, so the next time that particular alien life form has the audacity to transgress on the bundle of cells that is you, you'll be ready.

The intruder is on file. You're preprogrammed to produce the appropriate antibodies and killer T cells. You can act fast to build the required army, and you have "acquired" immunity to that particular pathogen. You acquire this immunity as you age, one disease at a time, which is why children are often ill as their bodies develop adapted responses each time a new pathogen comes along.

Killer T cells attack with perforin and granzyme much like natural killers. The difference is that killer T cells are simple-minded assassins. They are built to respond to only one antigen, and when they find that particular chemical signature displayed on a cell membrane, they kill first and don't know how to ask questions later. This is the Achilles' heel of the acquired immune system: killer T cells ignore invaders, no matter how deadly they might be, that do not display the appropriate antigen.

If you could brand cancer cells with a chemical marker, and train killer T cells to attack that marker, then you could theoretically kill that cancer. Many factors, including the ability of mutants to evolve quickly, complicate such a cure to cancer, yet research progresses along these lines. It may be that one day the acquired immune system will be able to identify and eliminate solid tumors, but until that happy day arrives innate immune cells remain your best internal bet against cancer.

Your battles against intruders are waged at the site of infections or infestations, but the war is also fought on the immune system's home turf, mainly in the spleen and the lymph nodes. The cellular advantage to fighting battles on immune turf is that the infrastructure to manufacture the machinery of war is close at hand. All cellular branches of the immune army are in close proximity, which facilitates the high degree of chemical communication necessary to expunge pathogens.

The fist-sized spleen is the largest organ in your immune system. It neighbors the left kidney, and is your main immune armory. In Chinese medicine, a fundamental connection is made in qi flowing from heart to spleen, and it is perhaps no coincidence that a dedicated artery delivers blood directly from the heart to the spleen, where it runs a concentrated gauntlet of all the various immune cells.

Intruders in the blood are identified, dispatched, and digested. Game, set, match—all in one organ.

The nodes in your lymph system are a second important repository for immune cells, where lymph is the thin liquid that remains after blood flows through tissues. There is a yin and a yang to it, because blood and lymph constantly cycle from the one to the other, and lymph flows through vessels that eventually recycle it back to the blood in the veins leading to your heart.

Lymph is pumped by the actions of your muscles, and couch potatoes take note. Nobody wants stagnant lymph. Backed up lymph is like a swamp where your enemies can fester. It's just one more reason to exercise, and lymph, as it trickles slowly through the lymph system, encounters lymph nodes.

Lymph nodes are capsules segmented with baffles that slow lymph flow even further, are concentrated toward the groin and neck, and come packed with immune cells that inspect the identities of cells in the passing fluid. Blood pumped by the heart moves through the spleen quickly. Some intruders invariably slip through, but the immune cells in the lymph nodes have the luxury of a leisurely examination.

Credentials can be scrutinized more closely, and imposters can be reduced to their constituent bits. The "swollen glands" in your neck and crotch when you get sick are evidence of lymph nodes at work. There's a fight going on. As an everyday average perhaps half of the fluid components of your blood filter through the lymph system, and, at first glance, it seems an odd place for cancer cells to lurk.

The lymph system is a well known highway for the spread of cancer, yet it is also immune system central. It doesn't make sense. What's going on?

The first problem is that, depending on the part of the body, it is possible for cancer cells to travel the lymph for varying distances, and then exit into hospitable tissue, without encountering a lymph node. Second, the acquired immune response only works on cells that present specific evidence of another identity, and many years of experiments have shown cancer cells to be fairly adept at not presenting antigens that would get them killed by the acquired immune system.

It's what you'd expect of a cell that once was you. On the other hand, as it becomes less and less like you, it makes fewer and fewer of the proper identifying offerings at the altar by which it is judged. It may not be making the wrong identities that will get it killed by the acquired immune system, but it may not be making enough of the right identities that will keep it alive when questioned by members of the innate immune system either.

Natural Killer Cell: "Your papers, please..."

Cancer Cell: "Here's an old bank statement...I must have something else..."

Natural Killer Cell: "Too late."

Mutant cells have to prove to natural killers who they are, not just who they aren't. Natural killers are at the forefront of your body's war on cancer, and it is therefore unfortunate indeed that these cells decrease markedly in abundance as the human body ages. Just when you need them most, you don't have them anymore.

It's not just natural killers. The entire immune system simply deteriorates over time. The immune army shrinks until you can't adequately staff the gates, at which point your lymph nodes have become like the Tijuana border crossing during rush hour. The guards are overwhelmed, and it's easier for the bad guys to slip through.

As you age there are more mutants and fewer inspectors. While a natural killer cell is inspecting the papers of one cancer cell two more mutants might be sliding by. The all-volunteer army is no longer working. What your immune system needs is a boost to recruitment, particularly in the ranks of natural killers, and many experiments show the chemicals in several plants, including echinacea, goldenseal, ginseng, and astragalus, apparently induce just such a recruiting boost.

Echinacea is a good example of the potential power of these plants because it is both well studied and highly consumed. The echinacea plant, prairie coneflower, is native to the North American plains, and was used for medicinal purposes by Native Americans since before Europeans arrived. Again, this is a drug that has been tested for hundreds of years on all kinds of people, including the sick, rather than a few months on a relatively healthy study group. Even so, very few people in the modern scientific community believe echinacea, or any of the plants mentioned in the previous paragraph, actually enhance the human immune system.

There is, however, a large body of modern evidence demonstrating the immune-stimulating properties of these plants, beginning with the chemical pathways through which they might work. For instance, in vitro and in vivo experiments indicate echinacea contains several potentially active ingredients, including cichoric acid, arabinogalactans, and alkamides. Structurally, these chemicals are very diverse, yet it appears they have the ability to act in a complementary manner on the human immune system.

Critically, the effect of the whole is much greater than any individual part.

Arabinogalactans are highly branched, dense, heavy carbohydrates with atomic numbers reaching into the tens of thousands. These sugars aren't just complex, they're very complex, and when digested by macrophages, induce the macrophage to send out the chemical call for more natural killers to be produced in the bone marrow.

At the same time, fatty molecules called *alkamides* inhibit levels of chemicals that are in turn meant to inhibit levels of natural killer cells. Inhibiting the off-switch is like increasing the on-switch, and the net result is that alkamides act to sustain any increases in the production of natural killer cells that arabinogalactans might provide.

Meanwhile, *cichoric acid,* the aromatic electron donor behind the distinctive tang of chicory, participates in chemical chain reactions that call for more macrophages. More macrophages digest more arabinogalactans, the call goes out for more natural killers, and the resultant high population of natural killers is encouraged by alkamides.

All that, neatly packaged in one inexpensive plant.

The effect on the immune system of the mutually reinforcing chemical spiral of echinacea has been tested in mice, both young and old, and sick and healthy. Five years of comprehensive research on the effects of commercial echinacea supplements on these mice were summarized in a 2005 review, and a couple of the early findings shed light on the larger issues of diet and dietary supplements as a whole.

First, researchers found medicines derived from whole plants more effectively stimulated the immune system, as opposed to medicines made from only roots or only flowers. Again, good diet isn't any one thing, it's a little bit of everything.

Second, researchers found eating echinacea improved the immune response in mice, but only up to a point. After that eating more echinacea didn't help. Appropriately, prorated by weight, that plateau dosage was roughly equivalent to what the product used in this study recommended for people, and, again, the larger point is that too much of anything is too much for you because there are no magic bullets.

As far as the actual effect of echinacea on young healthy mice, whole extracts of high quality plants administered at adjusted recommended dosages over a two week period stimulated the number of natural killer cells in the bone marrow and spleen by more than 25 percent. Monocytes, the precursor cells to macrophages, were also about 25 percent more numerous in young healthy mice receiving supplements. While levels of these innate immune cells rose, researchers found that levels of the various cells associated with acquired immunity remained relatively constant.

The scientists next tested the effects of echinacea on old healthy mice. These are like baby-boomer mice, with immune systems that have degraded over time. Just like me, they need help, and in old healthy mice two weeks of dietary echinacea increased the number of natural killer cells in the spleen by about 30 percent, up to the levels of young adults. Natural killers in both aging mice and aging humans tend to lose potency, but this study also noted an enhanced killing capacity, again to the levels of young adults.

Talk about a fountain of youth.

Even among health practitioners who recommend echinacea as a dietary supplement there is disagreement on the dosing regimen. One camp believes echinacea should be taken long term on a daily basis for proactive disease prevention, while a second camp believes chronic use builds up a resistance to the effects of the drug, and that echinacea should be taken only when a person feels sick. There hadn't been much experimental evidence either way, so these same researchers got mice hooked early.

In this experiment inbred (genetically similar) mice were fed a daily dose of echinacea beginning at puberty in week 7 and continuing until the beginning of "old age" at thirteen months. The echinacea mice were then compared to similarly inbred control mice who received the same diet in the same conditions with the sole exception that they did not get echinacea. At ten months the control mice had a 79 percent survival rate; all the echinacea mice were alive. At thirteen months 46 percent of the control mice were alive, while 74 percent of the echinacea mice were alive, and the researchers concluded that daily use did indeed confer enhanced long term immunity, at least in inbred mice.

This conclusion was supported by significantly higher absolute numbers of natural killer cells in the echinacea mice at every sampling period over the course of the experiment. Natural killers were more prevalent both in the bone marrow (where they originate) and the spleen, and since natural killers are naturally tough on cancer, the researchers next tested the effects of echinacea on cancerous mice.

Mice, with no say in the matter, were injected with a dose of leukemia known to consistently result in death 3.5 weeks later. Following injection some mice got echinacea, some didn't, everything else about diet and habitat was the same. At nine days the number of natural killer cells in the echinacea group was "very significantly" larger. At three months of age, long after all the control mice were dead, the levels of natural killer cells in the surviving mice of the echinacea group were more than twice as high as levels in normal mice of the same age, gender, and genetics.

Astonishingly, in these mice that had been given a death sentence, about one-third of them went on to live full mouse lives, while microscopic examinations at three months were unable to find any remaining cancer cells. In essence, it appears echinacea cured their cancer, most likely by stimulating production of natural killer cells. You have to be careful when comparing mice and men, but still…

Many studies have shown the concentration of active ingredients in echinacea varies significantly from plant strain to plant strain. Perhaps it would be possible to high grade for the good stuff, select for particularly effective plants, and fighting cancer could become as easy as pulling up to the window for takeout.

The whole super-size phenomenon is a paradigm of how not to eat, so in this more enlightened universe we'll call our fast food joint McAlboe's, where the letters in the name stand for "a little bit of everything." The mascot for this restaurant chain is a dancing cell, and because this universe is not so enlightened as to have grown past the need for marketing gimmicks, the employees are forced to dress as cells.

"Can I help you?" says the girl leaning out the window.

You can't help but admire her mitochondria, then you order:

"Let's see…I'll have the mini-burger, six fries, a large garden salad, echinacea dressing, and some natural killers to go…hold the trans fats and preservatives."

"Certainly sir…will there be anything else?"

Your wife, who dislikes the bitter taste of echinacea, leans over the console of your hybrid car and speaks toward the speaker phone. She's pushing sixty but she looks forty because she's been boosting her immune system all along, and she says what she always says.

"Hmm," she says, "I think I'll have the Chinese."

Ginseng contains dozens of active ingredients, and consuming this plant has been linked to stimulation of the innate immune system through macrophage activation and increases in natural killer number and potency. Another traditional Chinese medicine, astragalus root, has been shown to stimulate T cell production along with macrophages. Taken together, ginseng and astragalus put the chemicals in place to potentially stimulate both the innate and acquired immune systems, and these two plants have been prescribed for millennia in treatments of "spleen deficiencies" and the restoration of the overall condition of "insufficient qi."

Been feeling tired lately?

As far as human trials go, clinical studies that examine the anticancer potential of medicinal plants are few and far between. Some clinical studies have apparently shown some immune boosting and cancer fighting power in ginseng-ingesting groups as compared to control, but the bulk of the research into the immune-boosting effect of echinacea in human trials has been done in the area of upper respiratory infections.

As usual, the evidence is mixed.

On the one hand, a 2007 analysis in the prestigious journal *The Lancet* determined taking echinacea reduced the length of any given cold by one to four days, that it reduced the chance of catching a cold by 58 percent, and that echinacea taken in combination with vitamin C apparently prevented the incidence of colds by 86 percent. On the other hand, a 2005 article in the equally prestigious *New England Journal of Medicine* examined the effects of echinacea root extract on 339 volunteers who were voluntarily infected with rhinovirus, and the authors mince no words when declaring echinacea ineffective in treating colds in both short and long term use.

Again, well studied echinacea is a good example of a larger problem, which is that all plants are not created equally. With echinacea, three different species of the plant are used in commercial preparations, and each species contains different amounts and kinds of active ingredients. Health of plants, time of harvest, and the nature of processing (not all companies use the same parts of the plant) further exert profound influences on the proportions and quantities of the delicate molecules that actually make it from the original plant to your body.

It's nonstandardized medicine, and researchers in the rhinovirus study that found echinacea to be ineffective at treating respiratory ailments addressed this issue by making their own medicine. Three different processes on one lot of root from one species of plant were used to produce three different batches of medicine, which were then analyzed for different chemicals, including the three previously mentioned major active ingredients in echinacea.

One of the batches of medicine had large quantities of one active ingredient, another batch had large quantities of a second active ingredient, while a third batch had a medium amount of one chemical and a minimal amount of another. None of the three batches contained all three active ingredients, yet studies on mice had already shown the effect of any of these chemicals when taken apart does not impart nearly the same therapeutic value as these chemicals do when taken together.

The synergistic and reinforcing chemical interactions that together lead to increased numbers of natural killer cells are lost, and it's not surprising that these medicines as prepared had limited effect on people infected with rhinovirus. It is surprising these researchers didn't at least come up with medicine that contained all the known active ingredients before proceeding with an expensive experimental trial.

It's not something that would have slipped by Otto Warburg. To me, it's sloppy science and, while this study didn't convince me echinacea is ineffective as an immune stimulant, it did convince me the quality of the supplements we use matters.

Again, this is an example of a problem in the larger whole. That problem is truth in advertising in commercially processed foods no matter where they come from, and an independent testing laboratory found that only four out of eleven commercially popular echinacea brands contained what their labels said they contained. Some brands had no echinacea at all, about half listed the wrong species of plant, and more than half did not contain the declared amount of active ingredients.

Similarly, the active ingredients by weight in commercially prepared ginseng have been shown to vary as much as twentyfold from capsule to capsule. It's a hugely confounding factor in how we as consumers must interpret the data from studies on the beneficial effects of medicinal plants, and in this I'm reminded of the infamous O.J. Simpson murder trial.

There was plenty of evidence O.J. did it but, when highly paid experts got done wrangling, there was insufficient proof. Similarly, there is plenty of evidence certain plants have certain healthful effects but, when highly paid experts get done wrangling, there is no proof. Even so, that doesn't mean O.J. didn't do it, and that doesn't mean these plants don't work.

At the very least, they're more affordable than health insurance.

As for me, I spend the extra five bucks it takes to get good echinacea, and I get it from a health food store where somebody I trust has already done the research to make sure the products are of high quality. I believe echinacea works because I understand the chemical pathways by which it might work and, when a person believes in a treatment, no matter what the treatment, another compelling body of research shows that treatment is much more likely to work.

Which brings us back to the brain.

It Doesn't Matter
What You Believe,
As Long as You Believe

Can the mind stimulate the immune system?

I guess it depends on whether you think rats have minds.

That the mind might affect the immune system was accidentally brought to the attention of western researchers in a 1974 experiment originally designed to study how long conditioned rats would remember an illness-induced taste aversion. In this test thirty rats were given 1, 5, or 10 milliliters of water sweetened with saccharine, followed thirty minutes later by a toxic agent that created "temporary gastrointestinal malaise."

That must have been some malaise because every rat associated sweet water with sickness after only one exposure, as measured by their reluctance to consume sweetened water over the ensuing days and weeks. The experiment found conditioned aversion was strongest in rats receiving the largest initial dose of sweetened water, and that the conditioned response proved quite resistant to extinction.

The rats, unfortunately, did not prove quite so resistant to extinction.

It was fifty days before conditioned rats were again drinking as much sweetened water as control rats, but at only forty-five days the conditioned rats began dying. It was a completely unexpected result, since if one-time gastrointestinal malaise could kill, we'd all be dead. Researchers had their first clue to the mysterious nature of the deaths when further evaluation of the chemical eaten by the rats revealed that, in addition to inducing gastric distress, it also suppressed the immune system.

Follow up research showed that rats, after a single exposure to this chemical, were associating not just nausea, but also the immune-suppressing effects of the chemical, with sweetened water. The subsequent taste of sweetened water was enough to cause the rats to suppress their own immune systems, and the rats learned the association so well that after only one lesson they were killing themselves.

Rat brains are one thing, human brains another, and this rat research led to a study on women receiving chemotherapy for breast cancer. Chemotherapy suppresses the immune system, and researchers found women arriving at the hospital for regular treatments, before receiving treatment, in response to what their bodies associated with what their minds knew was coming, suppressed several important indicators of immune function at the mere sight or (perhaps) smell of the treatment center.

In another study ten patients with an autoimmune disease (multiple sclerosis) were conditioned to associate anise flavored syrup with a drug that inhibited immune response; eight out of ten patients showed diminished immune response in response to the syrup alone in a magnitude similar to the effects of the actual drug. Subsequent studies showed this conditioning affected immune cell numbers, along with several chemical messengers in the immune response.

Most researchers attribute this immune suppression to classical conditioning, or an innate response to a learned stimulus. Pavlov's dog learned to associate food with the ringing of a bell, and ringing the bell (a learned stimulus) then caused the dog to drool (an innate response). Classical conditioning is thought to occur independently of conscious expectation, and because of this, conventional wisdom has long held you'd be better off washing the drool off your dog than attempting to consciously boost your immune system.

This view is changing as research finds that the distinction between conscious and unconscious thought might not be quite as vivid as was once thought. Conscious expectation may not be necessary for a conditioned response to occur, but that doesn't mean conscious thought can't affect innate functions. To the contrary, many studies show people consciously alter innate functions like heart rate and respiration, and many more studies link conscious thought with changes in innate immune function through the parameter of stress.

Stress is hard to measure because it's different things to different people. Fear and anxiety in the face of an unpleasant threat are involved, but not all people find the same things unpleasant. It helps if you feel you have control of the situation, it hurts if you don't, and recent research distinguishes between the acute stress of getting held up at gunpoint and the chronic stress of getting divorced.

A 2004 meta-analysis of over three hundred papers on the effects of psychological stress on the human immune system found acute, brief, and chronic stress manifested in different ways. Acute stress is the response of our bodies to immediate peril. It can be measured by how well you survive life-threatening situations, but in experiments acute temporary stress is approximated by parameters such as public speaking or mental math. Slightly longer but still brief stress is usually measured in students taking tests, while the effects of chronic stress are generally strongest in people who suffer a blow to their identity, something like losing a job or living with a newly acquired handicap.

Obviously, the acute stress of trying to multiply 27 times 27 in your head pales in comparison to the acute stress of going looking for firewood and finding a saber-toothed cat instead. The causes of stress are far different than they were. In the old days, when you came upon a saber-toothed cat, you got scared, and scared is good, because it triggers a rapid body-wide response to that stress.

Electrons flow in the sympathetic nerve fibers that directly connect the brain and the bone marrow, thymus, spleen, and lymph nodes. Recent studies show the net effect of acute stress is to increase the activity of the innate immune system and decrease the activity of the acquired immune system. It takes time and energy to clone an army of T cells; energy is instead diverted to making and delivering more innate quick responding cells like natural killers to peripheral tissues where wounds are likely to occur.

In response to a stressful emergency the chemicals adrenaline and cortisol flood your blood, triggering a cascade of chemical messengers that activate three of your body's primary feedback loops. The sympathetic nervous system, the brain stem, the hypothalamic, pituitary, and adrenal glands, and the sex organs are all involved in mounting an integrated response to get you fired up for action. It's a lot to go through just to prepare for a speech in front of some strangers you'll probably never see again.

The response is more appropriate to our animal past, where you'd run if you could, but the saber-tooth cat has already seen you. You're not going down without a fight. You blow into your bone horn, summoning help while you unsheathe your flint knife. You're taking control of the situation. You're not going to let stress get the better of you. You're not going to panic. You're going to think.

Then, as now, that's how you handle acute stress.

You use the rush to your advantage.

Continued stress is called brief rather than acute, and studies show that this slightly longer term stress induces the production of a chemical that informs helper T cells to prepare to fight pathogens outside the cell as opposed to inside the cell. The immune system prepares to deploy forces on a larger battlefield and in the old days that was it. You either got yourself a new lion skin coat or you got yourself eaten.

Tastes like pork, or so the cannibals say.

One way or another, it was over. You fired up in response to a stressful situation but, no matter how dire the emergency, you can only stay fired up for so long. Plus, no matter how powerful your will might be, you can only fire up so many times. It takes energy to mount an immune response, and if your body keeps answering the call to stressful arms, and the stress doesn't go away, after a while the effect on your immune system is like the boy who cried wolf.

The townspeople quit responding in a concerted manner. They can answer the call like they mean it only so many times before they lose interest. Chronically elevated levels of cortisol and adrenaline affect your entire being, including such basics as the ability of your hippocampus to form memories. The meta-analysis of the effects of stress on the immune system found that chronic stress diminished every measured aspect of the immune response, including very substantial decreases in the numbers of killer T cells and the potency of natural killers.

It's an unhealthy mix because hit men from both sides of the immune family are compromised in their ability to do their jobs. This across the board decrease in immune function was seen in young and old, and in men and women. The cumulative effects of chronic stress certainly play a role in the well documented decrease in immune function with age, and it is no surprise that studies show beginning at about age fifty or so people who have been under long term chronic stress are more vulnerable to disease.

Stress kills, there's no doubt about it.

But what about the flip side of the coin?

Chronic conscious stress negatively affects the immune system, but can positive conscious thoughts positively affect the unconscious immune system? If you're fighting cancer, can you think yourself into increasing your levels of natural killer cells? It seems farfetched, yet there are mounds of evidence that conscious thoughts can have huge beneficial effect on unconscious pain.

This is the placebo effect, and recent studies have begun to broaden the conventional view of this phenomenon. For instance, a 2008 comprehensive review of the placebo effect reports that "The focus has shifted from the 'inert' content of the placebo agent (e.g., starch capsules) to the concept of a simulation of an active therapy within a psychosocial context."

In other words, it's not the pill that does the work, it's the mind.

This may seem obvious but for decades it wasn't. As an example of the dogma over those years consider the hypothetical trial of a new prescription drug. Again, these numbers are hypothetical, yet not atypical of actual results when a new drug is approved. In this hypothetical trial suppose the drug helped 70 percent of the patients who tried it, while a placebo helped 50 percent of the people, and meanwhile in the control group 40 percent of the people showed improvement without any treatment at all.

Results like these are generally interpreted to mean the placebo didn't work, because it did not perform significantly better than the control group. To me, this misses the whole point of placebo, which is that (when averaging many studies) you find one-half to one-quarter of patients improve using nothing more than their minds.

A true control group for a placebo would consist of patients that did not want to get better, a group that generally does not exist. Comparing two groups that want to get better is like comparing a blue sugar pill to a yellow sugar pill and concluding that because neither color worked significantly better than the other that neither color worked. It's a counterintuitive view that is changing rapidly, and in the last few years several experiments have been designed to measure how consciousness in the form of expectation, desire, and mood might affect treatment outcomes.

Expectation, as a manifesting factor in the placebo effect, was measured in a series of studies on the "open-hidden" paradigm. In this experimental technique some hospitalized patients are openly administered a drug. They're told they're receiving the drug and that they can expect relief from it. Another group of patients receives the same amount of the same drug, except they're not told that they're receiving it. It's just added to their intravenous solution without their knowledge.

In one such experiment five commonly used pain relieving drugs, including morphine, were studied. No matter what the drug, declared pain relief was higher in all five of the groups receiving the drug in an open fashion, and by a remarkable factor of two to three times the amount of reported relief. Follow-up variations on the open-hidden experimental theme led the reviewers in the 2008 paper to conclude that open administration of a drug is significantly more effective than hidden administration, and "conscious expectation is necessary for placebo analgesia."

The nuances of the effects of that conscious expectation were studied in another experiment, this time using patients with irritable bowel syndrome who were exposed to rectal distension by means of a balloon barostat. I know what you're thinking. A balloon up the butt, it's no wonder their bowels were irritated. It seems like a study better left to the rats, but these people volunteered.

One group of patients was instructed that they "may receive an active pain reducing medication or an inert placebo agent." This group was then treated with either medicated cream or a placebo, and then each of these subgroups was compared to a "natural history" unmedicated control group. In this experiment, in which patients knew they might be receiving a placebo, medicated cream performed significantly better than placebo, and placebo performed significantly better than control.

A second study was conducted in similar fashion, except no mention was made of placebo to patients, even though that's what some of them got. Instead, in a carefully worded statement deemed ethically acceptable, all patients were told the "agent" they had been given was "known to significantly reduce pain in some patients." In this trial, the placebo group experienced nearly the same pain relief as the medicated cream group, and researchers concluded overt suggestion may raise placebo analgesia to a magnitude matching that of an active agent.

If you expect a treatment to work it is more likely to do so, and other studies indicate desire and mood similarly influence the placebo effect. Simply put, you are more likely to get better if you expect to get better, want to get better, and are having a good as opposed to a bad day. Other studies show the placebo effect will most likely manifest in people who have an obtainable goal, and the magnitude of overall placebo relief is best explained when the combined results of desire and expectation are multiplied rather than added together.

That's not such a tough pill to swallow.

Expect your treatment will work, work toward a goal, want to get better, and have a laugh now and then, and health benefits don't just add up, they multiply. If you put it all together, with an eye toward how your mind might be an ally in your battle with cancer cells, you might begin with the goal of increasing natural killer cells.

You're tired of cancer cells roaming your lymph with impunity. You're going to fight back against metastasis. You're going to ramp up the number of guards in the gauntlet that cancer must run, and one way you might do this is by eating high quality echinacea that contains a blend of molecules that can work together to provide sustained increases in your number of natural killer cells.

It helps me to know how these molecules work, because then I'm more likely to believe that they will work, and if I believe they work, then they're more likely to work. It's a positive feedback loop, but it doesn't stop there. Hundreds of books have been written about how to decrease stress in your life, and if you next follow the advice in any one of those books, then you're coming at the problem from both sides.

You're decreasing chemicals that inhibit your immune system, you're increasing chemicals that boost your immune system. The combination of factors is much more likely to increase your number of natural killer cells than either factor alone, and, since you believe it can work, it's that much more likely to work. The benefits of belief multiply, and, conversely, so do the detrimental effects of negative thoughts.

If you're taking a long term medication you're not sure of, wash down meals of refined flours moist with partially hydrogenated oils, and stew about how the neighbors have a bigger television than you do—well, those effects also multiply.

It all comes down to belief, and measuring the effect of belief is like trying to capture the wind or precisely locate an electron. Belief is flux. It changes from one person to the next, it changes within the same person from one moment to the next, and different people believe in different things. The act of measuring belief affects the final measurement, and by the time you finish the measurement, what you've just measured is already something else.

So how do you measure it?

The simplest experiments are the best, and in one creative study on the effect of belief, patients recovering from heart attacks were given a picture of a heart. On that piece of paper, the patients were asked to diagram how much damage they believed their hearts had sustained. The researchers found that, regardless of the actual amount of damage any given heart had sustained, the size of the damage those patients sketched in on those pictures proved to be a more reliable indicator of functional recovery and future health care costs than did the standard blood test usually used.

In other words, the people who believed they didn't have a big problem didn't have a big problem, no matter how big their problem really was. They had faith they would get better, and, as a further example of the power of belief, other studies indicate that people with a strong spiritual faith tend to have stronger immune systems and recover more quickly from illness or surgery than nonbelievers.

Philosophers and theologians have long argued the biological purpose of religion, and one prevailing wisdom is that religion developed as a social constraint that made it easier for people to live together without killing each other. However, it is also possible faith is an evolutionary trait, based not on social advantages that make it easier to establish peaceful societies and reproduce, but on medical advantages. If you were a believer, perhaps you were more likely to live. Perhaps your body was more likely to heal itself than were the bodies of those other pagan hominids.

Maybe that's why our cousins the Neanderthals died out.

We'll never completely understand the interplay of mind and matter, but we do know conscious thoughts affect the workings of our more primitive nervous system as measured by factors such as pain or immune function. The chemical pathways are there. The evidence in human trials is there. Your thoughts can do good, and your thoughts can do bad, yet most doctors disregard the idea you can consciously increase your number of natural killer cells as uninformed or inappropriately optimistic.

As far as uninformed goes, we're back to the difference between evidence and proof, and concrete, repeatable double-blind proof will always be difficult to come by when measuring something that changes from moment to moment, like a mind. As far as inappropriate optimism goes, the idea here is that patients who don't get better might blame themselves for not trying hard enough, but to me that's like saying you didn't give it your best shot, because you knew you might fail.

There's nothing wrong with failing.

We all have to go sometime. It's just the way it is. I'd prefer to go knowing I'd done everything I could, as opposed to making excuses at the Pearly Gates where Saint Peter peers down over the top of his gilded scroll.

Saint Peter: "You're early."

The kids, the job, the bills, the sitting in front of the television—you knew you hadn't been taking care of yourself, but you figured all those pills would make up for it.

You never thought it would come to this.

You: "Well...I've been busy."

Saint Peter, after two thousand years of checking people in, has heard it all, and is not above a little sarcasm.

"Is that grease stain on your necktie from a doughnut or a french fry?"

The Pearly Gates gleam behind Saint Peter, but he jerks a thumb off to the side.

"Follow that path."

So, if faith matters, where do we go…

I Fish Therefore I Am

For me, it's a trout stream.

The best things don't come easily, so the fish aren't just big, they're tough. It's a part of Heaven where the angels have all pawned their harps for guitars and fiddles and such, and gather in bands as they wait for the evening rise.

The music tends toward Grateful Dead-ish extended jams since, no matter how many songs you know, eternity is a long time. It can all get to be so much that after a while you just have to take a break, so somebody wanders over to the creek to turn the water into wine.

Now all God's creatures, including the fish, are happy.

Excluding the alchemy, for a couple months, I had that Heaven on Earth.

If I was checking out I was going to pack it in before I left, and in the months following my radiation I played music most days, but I fished every day. Mostly I went high in the mountains above my house, where the river was small, the trout wild. The country is a hundred variations on the word beautiful, it's also useful.

Local trees include pine-needled larch, oozing sap sweet with arabinogalactans, the same dense complex carbohydrates found in echinacea. The wildflowers are thick on the banks, white yarrow and purple coneflower, blue flax and self-heal, just a few of the many medicines Native Americans have been using for millennia.

In the river above my house high water in the spring washes the inside bends free of willows, leaving open cobbled flats. These areas that open from river to sky aren't huge, but there's room for a back cast. In some bends it's fun just to cast, but in others you might want to creep, on hands and knees across the gravel, coming in low to the deepest pools, which hold the largest fish.

These are predatory brown trout, first imported from Europe just over a century ago, and now grown fat on silver slivers of baby native cutthroat trout. These are wild trout, smart and aware. If you alert them to your presence it's over. Even a single false cast can spook them, but if you crawl up, so close you can extend the rod and simply drop a grasshopper fly on the water, then you just might have an up close and personal encounter with an animal that traces its lineage back half a billion years.

Some fish you never forget, one of mine came from a pocket carved into a bank where the river is undercutting an old-growth fir. The huge tree is beginning to lean, and exposed roots dance where they dangle into the current. The fish was half as long as my leg, with red spots the size of dimes, taken so close it soaked me with spray as it soared in shaking leaps, and if that isn't Heaven, it's at least on the same street.

It's the same idea with a different address, and as I fished that summer I came to a view of paradise that was the first I'd ever really believed in. It's the idea that whatever it is, we've already got it. It's the knowledge that we're already part of a greater spiritual whole, and the crux is water, the spark of life.

About as soon as Earth's crust cooled enough to keep water from boiling we had oceans, and about as soon as we had oceans we had life. It's amazing really. Our planet likely coalesced into relatively solid form about 4.5 billion years ago, while a couple lines of evidence put the age of the oceans at between 3.8 and 4.2 billion years, and the earliest fossils date back to about 3.8 billion years ago.

All that water back then, it's the same water today. The water in you, the water in me, we just celebrated our four billionth birthday. It's a vast wealth of shared experience, and nobody knows where it came from.

One popular theory to explain the tremendous amount of water on this planet involves a collision with an icy moon, and if life did come from outer space, it was a time rife with opportunity to hitch a cosmic ride. The planet was being bombarded with potential extraterrestrials as the solar system coalesced, but a lightning zap in a puddle of organic fatty acid molecules could just as easily have jump-started cellular life.

However life happened, it happened only once.

The conservation of certain cellular processes indicates that the miracle of using pigments to obtain energy from the sun, and then to use that energy to pull electrons from water, and then to store those electrons as energy for future use in the form of carbohydrates, was a miracle that was achieved once and only once.

At any rate, once formed, life proved to be quite tenacious.

Early Earth was riddled with volcanism, earthquakes, tsunamis, and impacts with comets, meteorites, and small moons. That's a lot to survive, and these simplest of original cells, prokaryotes, are very small and lack complex internal organelles. We tend to dismiss these primitive organisms from our lofty perch as people, but prokaryotes were not only here first, they'll likely be here last. Even today, there are tens of millions of these elemental cells in a gram of soil, half a million in a milliliter of surface ocean water, and an unimaginable 3.9×10^{23} prokaryotes in a healthy human colon.

That's a lot of company when you're doing your business.

As the eons passed Earth became a much less tumultuous home for life. A turning point came about 2.5 billion years ago, when, following a final burst of massive basalt lava flows, the continents stabilized. Stable continental shelves provided habitat for simple oxygen-producing cells called cyanobacteria to prosper, and for the next half billion years or so iron quietly oxidized in the oceans, oxides that precipitated out as the rust colored banded formations from which we get iron ore.

Only when all the dissolved iron oxidized did atmospheric oxygen begin to accumulate, and by about 1.8 billion years ago oxygen had rocketed (in geologic time) from near zero to about 15 percent of the free gases in Earth's air. This provided an energy source that would usher in the second great age of life on this planet, the age of algae.

Algae are eukaryotes, larger cells characterized not by just a single membrane but by membranes within membranes. The cell as a whole is bound by a membrane, but smaller membranes also define a distinct nucleus and distinct internal organelles. These internal organelles include mitochondria, the cellular power plants that process the oxygen that provides the energy that allows the cellular differentiation of membranes within membranes in the first place.

Cells needed to have energy to differentiate, and they needed to differentiate to have energy. Which came first, the chicken or the egg? In the case of complex cells it's likely the chicken came with the egg, because to this day mitochondria contain their own DNA, and it is thought these cellular powerhouses are the scavenged remains of some long gone species of energy-producing cyanobacteria that established symbiotic residence in another type of bacteria.

Think of it as the opposite of apartheid.

The similarity of mitochondria throughout the plant and animal kingdoms again points toward an evolutionary miracle that happened once and only once; eukaryotic cells represent the second and so far last great advance in cell design. From natural killers to neurons there are 210 unique cell types in the human body, each producing the distinctive blend of fats and proteins specific to its particular function, but all according to the basic eukaryote cell plan of membranes within membranes.

Cells create products, and an undifferentiated prokaryotic cell is like running a business out of a tiny garage where the same cluttered bench serves for construction, packaging, shipping, and bookkeeping. You can only do so much. Eukaryotic cells, on the other hand, are like having a dedicated manufacturing plant with departments in particular places with specialized personnel attending to specific tasks on dedicated machines. These cells are capable of comparatively prodigious amounts of production, but they require comparatively prodigious amounts of energy, an energy bill that is financed by free molecular oxygen that makes it possible to extract nineteen times more energy from a single molecule of glucose.

Oxygen makes complex cells possible, and, without oxygen, cells can't be complex. Fix your oxygen and you fix yourself. This is one lesson of our cellular past, a second is that as beings comprised of complex cells we're all in this together.

It doesn't matter whether you're an accountant or an oak tree or a sea slug; our cells all face the same challenges in staving off the universe. Figuring out new ways to keep the universe at bay is not an easy proposition, and, after algae ushered in the age of complex cells, it would be on the order of another billion years before early animals, soft-bodied hydra-like creatures, began to appear in the fossil record.

Animal life grew increasingly complex, and about 500 million years ago began growing hard protective bodies. At this point in time, all the basic body plans (or phyla) of life we see today were already represented. These cellular blueprints included an unprepossessing sea creature with a unique evolutionary advantage: a backbone protecting long neurons that allow electrochemical messages to be sent directly, not just from cell to cell, but from one part of an organism to another part of an organism.

This was the body plan of the first vertebrate, and thus began the age of fish. And later, the amphibians and reptiles who would try to eat those fish. And much later, the mammals who would try to catch those fish on tufts of feathers and hair, only to let them go, and, as I crept over the rocks on my hands and knees, I sometimes felt like so much a part of the larger whole that it was all I could do to keep from weeping.

With joy.

And sadness.

As far as summers of fishing went, odds were this was my last. I was determined to properly enjoy it, and each afternoon I fished the tiny twisting river above my house, where the water is small and intimate. I'd spent so many decades guiding out of a drift boat on the big famous rivers that I'd forgotten the sheerest glee of stalking a stream, and as I crept through the green and yellow willows the years peeled away.

I felt like a kid again, like I was seeing it for the first time as trout rose to inspect floating flies, and then twisted at the taste of steel in silver leaps to the blue sky. When I hooked those memorable fish, the big ones from up so close they soaked me with spray that was nearly as old as the planet, well then I would just laugh and laugh and laugh at my place in it all.

The earth and water around me teemed with single-membraned cells in numbers so vast as to be no more imaginable than the extent of space. Thin, green tendrils of algae, the earliest expression of the complex cells that excess atmospheric oxygen made possible, wiggled in the currents below the boulders. The leaping trout at the far end of my fly line manufactured molecules like cholesterol and cannabinoids that bridged the gap from complex plant to complex animal cells, while the gray-bearded fisherman at the near end of the line was simply a more intricate manifestation of the trout.

I believed, and because I believed, I felt like part of a greater whole. The ancient religions are usually based in some form of animism. The idea is that there isn't just one God, there are many, and each spirit looks after a different part of the Earth. Mountains, sky, rain, trees, flowers, animals, and us, we all share a common heritage that links us in ways we will never fully understand, and as I crept along the river, I felt not only that I belonged, but that I mattered.

I had faith.

Even a mile above sea level in the shadow of the continental divide the August afternoons can swelter, and sometimes I'd get hot too. Lack-of-testosterone-induced hot flashes plagued me all through those summer months, and I stumbled (literally) into the discovery that wallowing in a trout stream is a fine cure to the common hot flash.

Of course, that's more of that anecdotal evidence. To be sure of the effect of trout streams on hot flashes we'd have to apply for a grant to do a study.

Want to be part of the control group?

It's far better than getting packed in beer cans, and as I luxuriated in the icy water, hot no more, I'd take time to envision a golden turtle in my belly behind the button. The turtle glowed as it drew energy from the energy around me, and the tumor in my prostrate shrank in the face of that positive energy like a puddle on a hot day. I visualized a testosterone starved cancer withering from the roots inward to a dead dry stalk bombarded with mushroom clouds of radiation. Every day I consciously devoted attention to the death of the tumor within me, and while there's no telling how much good it did me, it did make me feel good.

I'd always told myself to live each day to the fullest, to live as if each moment was the last, and those summer days I thought might be my last were the best I ever did at simply existing in that moment. There were times when I felt as if my spirit actually soared, and I could look down from the clouds with the circling hawks to the river below, and there I would see myself, oddly enough, the happiest I'd ever been.

The End of the Beginning

So, cancer...

What do you do?

When I grabbed my last cookie and left that hospital, having absorbed enough X-rays to kill a cockroach, the unspoken implication was that everything that could be done had been done, and, that everything that mattered had been done within those hospital walls. Well, that's madness.

If I'd stopped there the odds were long I'd be dead right now. But I didn't stop. It felt like I was walking away from a fight that wasn't over. After all that radiation I was more at risk for cancer than I'd ever been. I didn't want to get sucker-punched when my back was turned, so I began the research that led to this book.

At first, the information was hard to believe. For instance, the National Institutes of Health reported white women in San Francisco get breast and uterine cancer at rates of 3,000 percent to 4,000 percent higher than rural populations in other parts of the world. Other data showed black men in Atlanta, Georgia get prostate cancer at rates over 10,000 percent higher than men who live in rural areas of China.

Ten thousand percent?

My conventional treatment was raising my odds about 1/500th of that.

Comparing these numbers is somewhat like apples and oranges. They measure different things, and certainly race and genetics matter, but the greater point is that western medicine may not even be the most important part of your treatment. Other factors play a huge role and can make all the difference in the world, which is the difference between life and death.

From the chemical perspective of our cells, what we eat and do to keep cancer from coming back is also what keeps cells from mutating in the first place. It's never too late to make changes that help your cells process energy more efficiently and, as anecdotal evidence I'm very happy to provide, I'm here to prove it.

Up until the time I was diagnosed with cancer my diet was pretty typical of most Americans. In retrospect I'd guess I got upwards of 15 percent of my calories from animal sources, up toward 40 percent from fats, and the rest in everything else. After a lifetime in a culture of hidden trans fat I was still eating my fair share, and Lord how I loved to wash it down with hefty chunks of good sharp prostate-pounding cheese.

I ate salads, vegetables, and whole grain bread. I ate some chocolate but never drank soda pop. Most days I walked three miles, up the road along the river and back, then I did some sit-ups and pushups. If asked, I would have reported a healthy lifestyle, but looking back, on a scale of ten to minus-ten, I give myself about a one.

I was doing some good things, but not enough of them. I was eating far too many bad foods, and all the exercise in the world can't make up for cell membranes plugged with fifty years of ongoing and accumulated trans fats. The good and the bad probably just about balanced out, which is both more and less than I can say about my head.

Cancer is a series of experiences, and one telling vignette for me came at a Christmas party after I'd been diagnosed but before I'd decided how to proceed. I was admiring the ornaments on the tree when the father of a friend approached me. I barely knew him, and hadn't known he'd had cancer, but when he said out of the blue:

"How didja get it?"

I knew exactly what he was talking about.

I just hadn't wanted to admit it to myself.

The cancer had been growing in me for a while before it was big enough to be felt by a probing finger. At the time that mutation took root I was in a deep blue funk, a relationship in shreds, broke again. On a mental scale of ten to minus-ten, I was minus-eight and swirling. My thoughts were dark, a repetitive black maelstrom, and by the time I got over it, I had cancer.

It's no wonder. A minus-eight for head-set and a plus-one for lifestyle adds up to minus-seven. I was making it tough on my cells. In contrast, at the time I was diagnosed, the love and support I received from family and friends was overwhelming. I got to go to my own wake. It was the best I'd ever done at living in the moment, so for a while there I'd have to say head-health-wise I was running at a perfect ten.

I was so happy I couldn't die, but it didn't last. I've slipped back some mentally. I'm no Zen monk. Enlightenment is fleeting in my experience, but I still do the turtle most days. I tell myself not to sweat the small stuff, I remind myself it's all small stuff.

I still walk, and now I'm swimming again. I eat far better, mostly by cooking with whole foods and avoiding processed foods when I eat out by ordering big salads. Without even trying, I lost all the weight I put on during testosterone deprivation, and then some. I'm within a couple pounds of what I weighed in college, not much of it sags, and, from, head to toe, I feel better than I have in years.

That's what cancer did for me.

It was a wake-up call, only this time I didn't just hit the snooze button.

Now, I'd give myself about a plus-seven for both lifestyle and head-set. I could do better, but I figure it's pretty good for someone born with a woeful lack of willpower. It's still a total of plus-fourteen, as compared to my earlier minus-seven, and the difference between positive and negative is the difference between getting paid and paying bills.

It's the difference between having money and owing money. It's your energy balance, and, mathematically, the difference between plus and minus is absolute. Positive effects multiply, as do negative effects. Good and bad can cancel each other out, so if you're serious about fighting cancer you have to get all the forces lined up.

For instance, no matter how positive your thoughts, they can't make up for molecules your cells need but don't get. No matter how well you eat, food can't make up for chronic stress. No matter how good your health insurance, it can't make up for poor nutrition and a festering mind-set.

It isn't one thing, it's everything.

There are no magic bullets, yet our airwaves are rife with advertisements for foods, drugs, and exercise videos that will work magic, if only you'll call in the next ten minutes. We know these products are good for us because it says so right there on the box, yet our country is buried under epidemics of cancer, heart disease, and diabetes. It doesn't make sense until you consider it in terms of an ancient Greek art form, the farce.

A farce typically features costumed actors in exaggerated situations, so we'll start with a doctor who is dressed for surgery even though he's on a game show set. His name is Doctor Doctor, the show is called "What's My Medicine?", and since television has pretty much become a medium of copycats, to save money we'll just recreate a real scene from a recently aired and very popular daytime doctor show.

In this scene, the goal is to select the snack food that is highest in antioxidants from three possibilities lined up on a table: popcorn, crackers, and baked potato chips.

Doctor Doctor: "On your mark, get set...go!"

Two women, in sensible skirts, high heels, and plenty of makeup, charge across the floor to select the snack they believe contains the most free-radical-neutralizing molecules. It's a race, and the winner is: "Popcorn!"

Doctor Doctor looks pleased, after all he's getting paid. The women in the race look sheepish, but they've earned it. An off-screen overhead monitor blinks "Applause," the audience cheers as instructed, and Doctor Doctor describes a recent study that found popcorn has high levels of antioxidants.

"More than some fruits..." here he pauses to wink, "...and veggies."

On cue, the audience cheers again.

"Popcorn, popcorn, he's our man;

If he can't save us, nobody can!"

It's possible you anticipated this result. Popcorn is not highly processed. It's heated up once, it pops. Popcorn is made from a whole kernel of grain, you'd expect it to have more nutrients. In fact, that was the larger message of the study Doctor Doctor didn't convey. Products made from whole grains had the highest antioxidant levels, while products made from refined flours had antioxidant levels approaching zilch.

So if you followed this sound-bite of medical advice, and started chowing down on popcorn to raise your antioxidant levels, you'd be doing yourself a lot of good.

Right?

Probably not.

Depending on the brand, popcorn has some of the highest levels of trans fat in commercially available food, as do a lot of whole grain crackers. And what exactly can pass as whole grain? Who knows. Not me, and I read the FDA definition for whole grain wheat, which is mostly about how much of a ground product will pass through sieves of different sizes. There are loopholes galore. If the two women in that race were truly serious about selecting a healthy food they should have turned away from that table full of commercially processed snacks and run like hell.

But then it wouldn't be a farce anymore.

And where's the profit in that?

"What's My Medicine?" is sponsored by companies who tout the healthful benefits of their processed foods, so some topics are taboo. You won't hear that the single best way to provide your cells with good molecules and deprive them of bad molecules is to avoid foods containing refined flours, processed oils, or simple sugars. The fact that this is pretty much everything in the grocery store is telling, and it wouldn't be possible if our farce wasn't government sanctioned.

Take soybeans for instance.

Food and drugs are the same as banking and the military. There's a revolving door between the top people in industry and the agencies that regulate those industries. It's cronyism that contributes to banking crises, seven hundred dollar toilet seats, and the fact that 93 percent of soybeans grown in the United States are now genetically modified, despite the fact that it has never been proven genetically modified organisms are safe either for people or the environment.

Soybean fields are now carpet bombed with a potent herbicide manufactured by the same company that brought us Agent Orange, and since the soybeans have been genetically modified to resist this herbicide, all the plants in the field die except the soybeans. This cuts down on weeding, which pumps up profits, especially for the company vending the necessary herbicide and the congressmen whose campaigns can then be financed. These genetically modified soybeans are then cracked, dehulled, run through magnets to extract iron, heated to over 150 degrees, chopped, soaked in the solvent hexane, degummed of phosphatides, alkali bathed to remove free fatty acids, filtered, bleached, evaporated, and, in the final bean indignity, hydrogenated at temperatures hot enough to break carbon bonds before being sold as cooking oil.

Now why wouldn't that be good for you?

Flax oil, anyone?

We all know flax oil is good for us. Right?

It says so right there on the box, but an episode of "What's My Medicine" we're not likely to see might be called "Fighting For Flax."

Doctor Doctor: "On your mark, get set...go!"

At the signal the Stimson family (Mom, Dad, Bart, and Lisa) begin to wrestle through a mud pit toward a low table containing flax oil gelatin capsules, flax seed crackers, and an open dish of ugly, brown oil. The goal is to select the product with the highest levels of polyunsaturated fatty acids, and the winner is "Ugly, brown raw oil."

"Ew-w-w," says Lisa.

"Don't have a plant, man," says Bart.

Dad eats all the crackers, obviously disappointed.

"Hey...you said there were gonna be doughnuts."

There is a huge difference between eating cold squeezed and cold stored oil of whole flax, and eating a gelatin capsule of filtered and fractionated oil that has been processed who knows how and stored at room temperature for who knows how long. The label on gel caps of fish or flax oil may tell you the easily destroyed molecules your cells require once were in those capsules, but that doesn't mean they still are. It doesn't even mean those molecules were there in the first place.

Research on echinacea, ginseng, and a host of other vitamins and supplements shows that these products rarely contain what they say they contain, and in many cases the differences are egregious. Some bestselling brands, when pulled directly from the shelves of our most popular drug stores, don't have any of the plants they say they have, others test out as capsules of pure starch.

Even if a vitamin pill actually contains vitamins, it doesn't mean swallowing it is going to do you any good. Those vitamins have to be absorbed to be of any use to your cells, and all you have to do is look at your urine after eating vitamin pills to know where those molecules are really ending up. Again, it's just common sense; when was the last time you peed bright orange or yellow after eating a salad?

Vitamin pills are no substitute for real foods that contain a whole spectrum of molecules developed in response to the same cellular dilemmas humans face. Raw foods will have more nutrients than canned foods, and canned foods more usable nutrients than pills. A highly processed hard vitamin pill that is brewed up in high temperature vats is less likely to have nutrients than a gel cap full of whole raw plant that has had no processing other than drying, grinding, and cold capping.

Processed foods are ubiquitous in our culture. You can't avoid them completely; all you can do is be selective. It's a matter of degree. The longer the list of ingredients you don't understand, the more likely it is to be bad for your cells. If the fine print says shortening, emulsifiers, or (partially) hydrogenated then you're getting trans fats even though the large print says you aren't. Enriched flours are simply refined flours with stray vitamins added and in no way compare with the nutritive value of whole grains, but even though the label says whole grain it doesn't mean it is.

There are as many loopholes in our labeling laws as there are in our tax code. It's impossible to figure out, so I compensate by buying my bread from a local bakery where the girls have hairy armpits and outfits carefully accessorized with second hand clothes. They're buying real whole grain flours, and the bread is being transported across town, not across the country. They don't need preservatives to maintain freshness. In a similar vein, just because some companies lie about what is in their pills and foods doesn't mean every company lies about their products. It comes down to a matter of trust, to common sense, and in this I rely on people who have done the research: my local knowledgeable experts, whether they're at the bakery or the health food store.

These products generally cost a little bit more, but that's because they're better. Organic soy milk may cost more, but if isn't sprayed it shouldn't come from genetically altered beans. It costs more to cold press, cold bottle, cold ship, and cold store raw flax oil. A pint can cost you twenty bucks, which is a lot until you compare it to the price of health insurance, or a disease like Alzheimer's.

Nobody knows what causes Alzheimer's just like nobody knows what causes cancer, but high energy brain and nerve cells require more highly unsaturated fatty acids than any other cells in your body. It's easy to see how nerves would be among the first cells to be affected by the lack of these molecules in a typical diet, and if nerve cell membranes lack the parts they need to provide oxygen for respiration, those cells can run cellular energy deficits. High energy functions become impaired, and Alzheimer's is a disease in which proteins produced by nerve cells are improperly folded, which results in a buildup of insoluble plaque rather than a soluble supply of usable molecules.

If cellular energy deficits due to improperly constructed membranes contribute to cancer; it's easy to see how cellular energy deficits could also contribute to the improper folding of proteins.

All those people lying in those hospital beds wondering who they are, maybe it's because they only thought their brains were getting the molecules they needed. After all, it said so right on the box. At this point all I have is my memories, so before I forget, I eat flax oil from sources I trust in combination with yogurt, which delivers easily digested lipoproteins directly to the cells that need them most.

This works for me but something else may work better for you. We're as different on the inside as we are on the outside. This isn't a diet book. Eat what you want.

You may want chicken instead of fish, or bacon on your burger. Anything goes, but if you limit yourself to on the order of four to six ounces of meat, cheese, and such each day, then you're getting about 10 percent of your calories from animal sources. A teaspoon or two of flax or fish oil, a couple tablespoons of olive oil, a tablespoon of butter (especially for cooking since the saturated fats hold up well under heat)—that's about 20 percent of your daily calories as a wide spectrum of fatty acids that your cells can use without a lot of extra effort to build healthy membranes.

That leaves 70 percent of your diet for fruit, vegetables, whole grains, and beans. It's a diet that is very likely to thwart the initiation, growth, and metastasis of cancer because it is a diet that is very likely to provide your cells with the parts they need to process energy in an efficient manner. It leaves open the whole world of tasty cooking, yet it is very likely to be very different than how you now eat, and that's the point.

This is something you can change.

Ten thousand percent differences in cancer rates between populations aren't the result of any one factor, yet most experiments measure one variable at a time. It's a big part of the reason there is so much conflicting health advice out there, and in an effort to account for this greater reality, some researchers lump these phenomenal differences in disease rates across populations under the causative heading of affluence.

So what's so bad about affluence?

As hominids, exercise is our heritage. Humans are designed to walk and climb, while the price many people pay for their affluence is eight hours behind a desk in a state of chronic stress. After working up a good road rage on the commute home they're too exhausted to cook whole food, so they spend their affluence on quick processed foods, and for exercise thumb the remote. The net result of these negatively reinforcing factors is that cells work harder to get less done, and when there isn't enough energy to go around cells malfunction in unpredictable ways, including cancer.

That's simple enough.

It's too simple really. It's hard to believe changing simple habits can make so much difference, until you look at it from the point of view of the individual cell.

Then it's the difference between life, death, and mutation.

Blind devotion to low fat processed foods does not provide your cells with the mix of nutrients they require. Simple sugars feed cancer. So do couch potatoes. Chronic stress impairs the immune system. If you don't believe you can get better, you're probably right, and the more of these factors you fix, the better off you're going to be.

It just made sense, and because it made sense, I actually did things to make life easier for my cells. I wouldn't have done it if I hadn't learned the science. For me, that's the first benefit of my research, because if I hadn't learned enough to convince myself to change my habits, I doubt I'd be the anecdotal evidence I am.

Not only am I still alive, I managed to emerge from the far side of radiation with the joyous pleasures of defecation, urination, and fornication relatively intact. Even if all my lifestyle changes did was help limit side effects it was worth it, and if I believe they also helped eliminate the cancer, then they probably did that too.

I had no idea what I would encounter on this journey of research, and what I found was hope. It was like health insurance without the premiums, and once I began to look at cancer in terms of how my cells processed energy then all my conventional and nonconventional treatments were swimming in the same pool. They could be compared, I could make informed decisions, and I didn't need a prescription to do it.

Of course, if you're swimming in the same pool with cancer, you're going to be scared. Fear is a poor position from which to make decisions, but whether it's cancer or heart disease, we're usually scared when we decide what to do. This fear often begins when concentrations of one chemical messenger or another in our blood are deemed to be either too high or too low. According to population-based studies this puts us at risk, and suddenly we're afraid to not do things about things that might not happen.

I accepted treatments and diagnostic procedures out of fear. I also felt guilty about things I didn't do that my doctors recommended I do, but I got over it, and that's something else I took from a cell-based look at health care. It's so simple even a fishing guide can understand it. It's simple enough that I can make my own decisions and, make no mistake about it, somehow you must sift through all the conflicting health misinformation and disinformation to make your own decisions.

For instance, my regular doctor thinks early detection is the best way of fighting cancer. It's tough to argue, after all, his finger found my cancer in the first place, and the smaller cancer is when you find it the better your chances of killing it.

On the other hand, every checkup he tells me my colon needs scoped, every checkup I tell him my nether regions have been violated enough for one lifetime. It's hard for him to accept that I would reject a procedure when the numbers say it saves lives, but the numbers also say unnecessary diagnostic procedures cost a lot of lives.

At this point in my life I'd just as soon eat a lot of fiber, avoid a lot of meat, squeeze my bowels with exercise, and believe I've upped my odds by addressing the cause rather than the symptom of the problem of polyps in the digestive corridors. Plus, my catastrophic health insurance wouldn't cover the cost of the procedure. By avoiding it, at the very least I'm able to spend what money I have left after paying my insurance on having some fun as opposed to discussing a photographic bowel exposé.

"Yep, looks good to me. I can see you've been eating a lot of fiber."

"No shit."

For me, once was enough. I wouldn't subject myself to cancer treatment again. When my time comes, it comes. It's OK. This was the argument that finally persuaded my doctor a colonoscopy was not right for me; unfortunately he's no longer my doctor, and I dread the thought of starting all over with a new one.

My old doctor can't do checkups and such because he joined a hospital staff. He'll make more money with less hassle and I don't fault him a bit. It's just that it points out a larger problem, which is that despite the documented and multifaceted beneficial effects of caring, long term doctor-patient relationships, caring, long term doctor-patient relationships are going the way of the dodo.

If you want to stay healthy in the twenty-first century, look in the mirror.

Now introduce yourself to your new medical chief-of-staff.

If you eat nutritionally complete foods, believe it matters, and would prefer to avoid an invasive diagnostic procedure, that's very different than eating prepared foods that are purported to be healthy, turning on the television so you don't have to think, and relying on pills to get your limp dick to rise. If that's the couch where your potato lies, augmenting frozen weight-watcher entrees with fifteen minutes on a treadmill and a handful of vitamin pills isn't much of a cancer deterrent.

Get serious about providing your mind and body with the basics they need to prevent the initiation, growth, and metastasis of renegade cells, and there's plenty of science that says what you do for yourself will be at least as effective as what conventional medicine does to you. Think of it not so much as beating the odds as improving them, and with every change you make, your chances of surviving without debilitating side effects just got that much better.

Cancer is an energy deficiency you can fight cell by cell in ways that restore energetic balances. It's a simple notion backed by over eighty years of research, and it doesn't get much press because helping you help yourself is much more likely to save your life than it is to contribute to the over two trillion dollars spent on medical care in the United States each year. We as individual patients can't change a world in which profit too often trumps health, but we can change our cells, and if enough of us change our cells maybe we can change the world, or at least the part of it we care about most.

That goes for you, Jason.

And you too, Stuart.

My sons.

Acknowledgments

I would like to thank Otto Warburg, who carried a medieval lance into a modern war, Johanna Budwig, who saw trans-fat-eating pigs turn blue, and Ancel Keys, who said, "diet fads are for the birds, if you don't like birds." These are my kind of people, except they're smarter, and it was a pleasure getting to know them through my research.

I would also like to thank all the musicians, artists, fishing guides, friends, and family who organized a fundraiser that made my experience with cancer much less financially onerous. All I can say is everybody should get to go to their own wake, and if you're ever in Helena spend some money at Miller's or the Blackfoot Brewery.

Thanks to my fellow writers who took time to read the evolving manuscript: Tom Harpole for insights and cheerleading, John Bayorth for road signs and mile markers, and the recovering hypochondriac Kate Chullova, who reminded me not to make it scary.

And finally, and mostly, my thanks to my wife Janet, without whom this book would not have been possible.

Notes

Listed below are the referenced works, and some references appear in more than one chapter. Web site URLs are current as of November, 2010.

WE HAVE MET THE ENEMY AND IT IS US

Walker, Richard, ed. 2002. *Encyclopedia of the Human Body.* New York: Dorling Kindersley Limited. 100 trillion cells, over 200 types, p. 14.

Earth to sun based on grains of sand approximately 1/16 inch diameter. en.wikipedia.org/wiki/DNA_repair — As many as 1 million cellular DNA lesions per cell per day.

Kolata, Gina. Oct. 27, 2009. Cancers can vanish without treatment, but how? www.nytimes.com/2009/10/27/health/27canc.html?_r=1 — Increasing evidence human organism can either fuel or squelch tumors.

Hanahan, D, and R. A. Weinberg. The Hallmarks of Cancer. *Cell* 100 (January 7, 2000): 57-70. Darwinian evolution, p. 57; self sufficiency in growth signals, p. 58; insensitivity to antigrowth signals, p. 60; tumor is mix of normal and cancerous cells, p. 60; acquired resistance to apoptosis, p. 61; alternative pathways to apoptosis that may be activated to kill cancer cell, p. 62; limitless replication potential, p. 62; acquired sustained angiogenesis, 100 microns of blood vessel, p. 63; metastasis cause of 90% of human cancer death, p. 65.

HUNG LIKE A CASTRATI

Grimm, P. D., J. C. Blasko, and J. E. Sylvester. 2003. *The Prostate Cancer Treatment Book.* New York: McGraw-Hill. Prostate gland specifics, p. 4-6; hormone therapy, p. 156-159.

www.pnhp.org/news/2010/september/number-of-uninsured-skyrockets-43-million-to-record-507-million-in-2009 — 2009, 50.7 million uninsured Americans. 2007, 25 million underinsured non-elderly adult Americans.

THE SPARK OF LIFE

Warburg, Otto. 1966. *The Prime Cause and Prevention of Cancer.* (AKA *Revised Lindau Lecture*) English edition by Dan Burk, National Cancer Institute.

en.wikipedia.org/wiki/Composition_of_the_human_body — Oxygen, 65%, carbon, 18%, hydrogen, 10%, by mass.

Periodic Table of the Elements. From protons to electrons, all things atoms.

Parker, Steve. 2007. *The Human Body Book.* New York: Dorling Kindersley Limited. Fats, phospholipids, proteins, cell membranes, and organelles, p. 26-27.

LESSONS OF THE LAKE

Baumann, P., W. Smith, and W. Parland. Tumor Frequencies and Contaminant Concentrations in Brown Bullheads from an Industrialized River and a Recreational Lake. *Transactions of the American Fisheries Society* 116, no. 1 (January 1987): 79-86. 44% of 4-year-old fish with liver tumors, p. 79.

FS-040, Lake Erie Water Quality: 1970's to mid 1980's. Ohio State University. Information on Lake Erie pollutants, p. 1-3.

Sharpley, A., T. Daniel, T. Sims, J. Lemunyon, R. Stevens, and R. Parry. Agricultural Phosphorous and Eutrophication. Agricultural Research Service, United States Department of Agriculture, Second Edition, ARS-149 (September 2003): 1-43. Phosphorous, algae, bacteria, oxygen and eutrophication, p. 1-2.

THE HORMONE EXPRESS

Parker, Steve. 2007. *The Human Body Book.* New York: Dorling Kindersley Limited. Hypothalamus size of sugar cube, p. 79.

Walker, Richard, ed. 2002. *Encyclopedia of the Human Body.* New York: Dorling Kindersley Limited. Dozens of hormones, p. 118-119; pituitary size of raisin, p. 122; pituitary produced hormones, p. 122-123; fever as immune response, p. 159.

For more on hypoxia inducible factor, see the later chapter on hypoxia.

Pert, Candace. 1997. *Molecules of Emotion.* New York: Scribner. Peptides and proteins, p. 64; peptide bonds boiled in acid to break down, p. 64; ligands and receptors, p. 24-27; agonist/antagonist, tamoxifen, p. 346; twenty common amino acids, p. 65; all steroids start out as cholesterol, p. 25.

LaBrie, F. Medical Castration with LHRH Agonists: 25 Years Later with Major Benefits Achieved on Survival in Prostate Cancer. *Journal of Andrology* 25, no. 3 (May/June 2004). "Completely unexpected scientific finding..." p. 305; in 2001 LHRH sales of 2.2 billion, p. 307; humans most sensitive to LHRH agonists, p. 305.

Casodex, bicalutimide tablets, AstraZeneca fact sheet 238848. Antagonist, p. 1.

www.ncbi.nlm.nih.gov/bookshelf/br.fcgi?book=cmed6&part=A15479 — Pharmacokinetics and metabolism; natural half-life of LHRH, 2-4 minutes; LHRH agonist half-life 7.6 hours, binding affinity 10 times greater.

Wilson, A. C., S. Vadakkadath Meethal, R. L. Bowen, and C. S. Atwood. Leuprolide Acetate: A drug of diverse clinical applications. *Expert Opinion on Investigational Drugs* 16, no. 11 (November 2007: 1851-1863.

A LESBIAN TRAPPED IN A FISHERMAN'S BODY

Howard, P. J. 2000. *The Owner's Manual for the Brain: Everyday Applications from Mind-Brain Research.* Austin: Bard Press. Female corpus callosum 23% thicker, p. 219; male brains wired to do, female to talk, p. 217; monkeys and testosterone, p. 219; rats and ovaries, p. 220; exercise increases endorphins, p. 157; stress shrinks hippocampus, p.391; chronic versus acute stress, norepinephrine, symptoms of stress, p. 387-391.

Astra-Zeneca, Manufacturer's Clinical Pharmacological Information, 238848, Casodex, bicalutamide tablets. Table 2, Incidence of adverse effects. 35% of patients reported general pain, 53% hot flashes; 22% constipation, 12% diarrhea, 52 categories of side effects reported in all.

LaBrie, F. Medical Castration With LHRH Agonists: 25 Years Later With Major Benefits Achieved on Survival in Prostate Cancer. *Journal of Andrology* 25, no. 3 (May/June 2004). Testosterone levels rise to four times normal then precipitously drop at 7-14 days, Figure 2, p. 307.

Shanafelt, T. D., D. L. Barton, A. A. Adjei, and C. L. Loprinzi. Pathophysiology and Treatment of Hot Flashes. *Mayo Clin. Proc.* 77 (2002):

1207-1218. Role of hypothalamus in hot flashes, p. 1208; epinephrine and endorphin interplay, p. 1209-1210.

Parker, Steve. 2007. *The Human Body Book.* New York: Dorling Kindersley Limited. Hypothalamus seat of chemical control, amygdala emotional seat, many nerves and chemicals intimately connect these two organs of the animal brain.

YOUR BRAIN VERSUS THE UNIVERSE

Freeman, E. The role of anxiety and hormonal changes in menopausal hot flashes. *Menopause* 12, no. 3 (May/June 2005): 258-266. Three and five fold increase in hot flashes linked to anxiety levels, p. 258.

Shanafelt, T. D., D. L. Barton, A. A. Adjei, and C. L. Loprinzi. Pathophysiology and Treatment of Hot Flashes. *Mayo Clin. Proc.* 77 (2002): 1207-1218. Raise endorphins, lower epinephrine to treat hot flashes, p. 1209-1210.

Nedstrand, E., K. Wijma, Y. Wyon, and M. Hammar. Vasomotor symptoms decrease in women with breast cancer randomized to treatment with applied relaxation or electro-acupuncture: a preliminary study. *Climacteric* 8, no. 3 (2005): 243-250. Exercise reduces vaso-motor symptoms, p. 2; relaxation technique, p. 3; results, Table 2, p. 5.

Wijma, K., A. Melin, E. Nedstrand, and M. Hammar. Treatment of Menopausal Symptoms with Applied Relaxation: A Pilot Study. *Journal of Behavioral Therapy and Experimental Psychiatry* 4 (December 28, 1997): 251-261. 73% symptom decrease, p. 251.

Evans, D. 2004. *Placebo: Mind over Matter in Modern Medicine.* New York: Oxford University Press. Fever as immune function, p. 49; Henry Beecher, p. 1-4; double blind clinical trial evolution and flaws, p. 6-14.

Nedrow, A., J. Miller, M. Walker, P. Nygren, L. H. Huffman, and H. D. Nelson. Complementary and Alternative Therapies for the Management of Menopause-Related Symptoms. *Archives of Internal Medicine* 166 (July 2006): 1453-1463. Five data bases yielding 1432 abstracts, p. 1454; data are insufficient to support the effectiveness of any complementary or alternative therapy, "little benefit...", p. 1453.

Shanafelt, T. D., D. L. Barton, A. A. Adjei, and C. L. Loprinzi. Pathophysiology and Treatment of Hot Flashes. *Mayo Clin. Proc.* 77 (2002): 1207-1218. 25% reduction in hot flashes with placebo, 1 in 5 has 50% reduction with placebo alone, 1 in 10 has reduction of at least 75% with placebo alone; antidepressant venlaxafine, 37%, 61%, 61% experienced relief at increasing doses of drug, p. 1212.

DOCTOR DILEMMA

Starfield, B. Is US Health Care Really the Best in the World? *Journal of the American Medical Association* 284, no. 4 (July 26, 2000): 483-485. 44,000 to 98,000 American deaths per year due to medical error, p. 483; 225,000 to 284,000 to error plus non-error medical procedures, p.484; third leading cause of death, p. 484; one study rates American health care at 12 out of 13 countries (next to last) on 16 indicators, another as 15th out of 25 industrialized nations, p. 483.

World Health Organization, World Health Report 2000, Annex Table 10, Health System Performance in all member states, WHO indexes, estimates for 1997. p. 200, 201.

Leape, L. Scope of Problem and History of Patient Safety. *Obstetrics and Gynecology Clinics of North America* 35 (2008): 1-10. 1.3 million to 15 million preventable adverse health events suffered by hospitalized patients, p. 1; iatrogenic issues under-reported for many reasons, p. 1.

Leape, L., and D. Berwick. Five Years After To Err Is Human. *Journal of the American Medical Association* 293, no. 19 (May 28, 2005).

THE SKINNY ON FATS

The Periodic Table of the Elements. All things atoms.

lipidlibrary.aocs.org/lipids.html — These sections, among other sections, are cited by page from the PDF downloads available at the end of each section:

What Is A Lipid? Definition, p. 1; tri-. di-, and monoglycerides, p. 2-3; cholesterol, p. 3; Table of various fatty acids by length of carbon chain and number of double bonds, p. 11.

What Lipids do. Polyunsaturated fatty acids important membrane constituent that decrease membrane rigidity, p. 2; interaction between saturated, mono-unsaturated, and poly-unsaturated acids necessary for correct balance between rigidity and fluidity, p. 3; primary function of cholesterol is to modulate membrane fluidity, p. 4; cholesterol ubiquitous component of animal tissues, p. 4; bi-layer is composed of amphiphilic phospholipids and cholesterol, insoluble proteins, p. 5; Docosahexaenoic acid (DHA) more flexible and compact (60% length of oleic acid), increases conformational disorder.

Fatty acids: Methylene-interrupted double bonds. Omega-6 lineoleic and omega-3 linolenic fatty acids, p. 1-2; arachidonic acid most abundant polyunsaturated fatty acid in phospholipids; omega-3 linolenic acid major component of leaves and photosynthetic apparatus; p. 3; soybean oil 7% omega-3, limits cooking value, p. 3; omega-3 important constituent of brain tissues, p. 3; DHA (22:6, n-3) reduce risk of colon cancer, p. 4; highly flexible DHA incompatible with rigid cholesterol creating lateral segregation and formation of rafts, p. 4; omega-3 and 6 formed in plants by insertion of double bonds in existing omega-9 fatty acids, p. 5; animal tissue only double bond between existing double bond and reactive carboxyl end, p. 6.

Phosphatidylserine and related lipids. 10-20% of phospholipids in cell membrane, 1; DHA leg, p. 1; n-3 to n-6 ratio higher in brain than other tissues, p.1; functions include assisting protein messaging through build-up of negative charge, activates key enzyme in signal transduction, important role in regulation of apoptosis, p.4; initiates mineral deposition in bone formation, p. 4; high concentrations in brain, p.4.

Cholesterol and cholesterol esters. Cholesterol ubiquitous in animal tissues, p. 1; comprise 30-50% of cell membrane, p. 1; brain contains more cholesterol than any other organ in the body, p. 1; amphiphilic, rigid, planar molecule that can interact on both sides, p. 1; span half-a-bi-layer, p. 2; function to increase membrane order, reduce passive permeability to solutes, p. 2; cholesterol can flip rapidly between leaflets in bi-layer, p. 2.

The battle over hydrogenation (1903-1920). There can be little doubt the goal to completely harden oils was for making soap, p. 1; Crisco released in June 1911, p. 4; massive advertising campaign including free cookbook with 615 recipes, instant success and economic and healthy alternative to butter, p. 4.

Commodity oils and fats-olive oil. Varied natural composition, p. 1.

Fatty acids: Straight-chain monoenic. Most abundant 16 or 18 carbons long, p. 1; cis-double bond creates 30 bend resulting in looser membrane packing, p. 1; omega- designation rules, p. 1; oleic acid most abundant monoenic fatty acid in plant and animal tissues, p. 2; ruminants produce trans fats, p. 2; other trans fatty acids rare, p. 3; plants use aerobic mechanism to insert double bonds in preformed saturated fatty acids p. 4.

FEAR OF FRYING

www.eatwisconsincheese.com/wisconsin/other_dairy/butter/butter
_basics/composition_of_butter.aspx — In 100 grams of USDA butter there are 51 g saturated fats, 31 g monounsaturated, 3 g polyunsaturated.

en.wikipedia.org/wiki/Trans_fat — History and nature of trans fat.

Crisco website: www.crisco.com/About_Crisco/History.aspx — Quote about Crisco not picking up odor of fish.

Sundram, K., A. Ismail, K. C. Hayes, R. Jeyamalar, R. Pathmanathan. Trans (Elaidic) Fatty Acids Adversely Affect the Lipoprotein Profile Relative to Specific Saturated Fatty Acids in Humans. *The Journal of Nutrition* 127 (1997): 514S-520S. Main fatty acid resulting from partial hydrogenation is trans 18:1, <2% trans-trans, p. 514S; negative effect of 18:1 fatty acids unmatched by other fatty acids, p. 514S; 5.5% intake of elaidic acid increases LDL/HDL ratio 40%.

Stender, S., A. Astrup, and J. Dyerberg. Ruminant and industrially processed trans fatty acids: health aspects. *Food and Nutrition Research* 52 (2008): 1654-1661. Trans fat in ruminant fat usually less than 6%, in milk trans fat is 4-6% of total fat. Greater than 20 g trans fat/meal in popular foods is possible, p. 1654; 5 g trans fats leads to 29% increased risk of heart attack, p. 1; trans 18:1 comprise 80-90% of total trans fat in human food, p. 1654; US mean intake of trans fat 5.3g/day, 90th percentile at 9.4g day; foods bought between 2005 and 2008 in US, large serving of nuggets and fries had 20 g trans fat, 100 g of cracker type products had 13 g trans fat, 100 g microwave popcorn had 15 g trans fat, Figure 3, p. 1656; negative effects include pro-inflammatory, pro-arrhythmia, and decrease in ratio of HDL to LDL.

Sun, Q., J. Ma, H. Campos, S. Hankinson, et al. A Prospective Study of Trans Fatty Acids in Erythrocytes and Risk of Coronary Heart Disease. *Circulation, Journal of the American Heart Association* 115 (2007): 1858-1865. Trans fats account for 2-3% of total US energy intake, p. 1858; 18:1 trans fats 70% of trans fats in erythrocytes, p. 1860; each 0.25% increase in 18:2 trans fat associated with adjusted relative risk of 2.2, while 18:1 associated with adjusted relative risk of 1.3, p. 1861; trans fatty acids alter membrane function and decrease fluidity, p. 1864.

en.wikipedia.org/wiki/Trans_fat — Wilhelm Norman patent in 1902; Crisco 1911; production of trans fat increased steadily through 1960's; 1988-1994 increasing evidence on detrimental effects of trans fats.

en.wikipedia.org/wiki/Polyethylene — Structure of polyethylene.

en.wikipedia.org/wiki/Great_Pacific_Ocean_Garbage_Patch — Estimates on the amount of plastic now floating in the Pacific Ocean.

www.fda.gov/Food/GuidanceComplianceRegulatoryInformation/ GuidanceDocuments/FoodLabelingNutrition/FoodLabelingGuide/ default.htm — Go to trans fats for Food and Drug Administration labeling requirements.

www.cancer.org/Cancer/CancerBasics/lifetime-probability-of-developing-or-dying-from-cancer — Statistics on cancer incidence.

BOUND BY THE CHAINS OF SCIENTIFIC DOGMA

First-hand accounts of the making of the Seven Countries Study are available at

www.sph.umn.edu/epi/history/sevencountries.asp — Addendum: Laboratory under Gate 27 at football stadium; differences between populations of coronary heart disease on order of five-to-tenfold; non-overlapping blood serum cholesterol of Japanese fishermen and Finnish Loggers; 3-22% variation in saturated fat, 9-40% variation in total fat; first study to apply partial correlation coefficients. Finland: "Loggers lunches are things of wonder..." Crete: walked or rode bikes, thyme scented fields, Overview: Central grant of $25,000 per year per country, surveys from 1958 to 1970 in 18 areas of 7 countries on men between ages of 40-59. Ancel Keys: Finns had heart attacks at rate of 992/10,000, while Cretans had heart attacks at rate of 9/10,000 people, "North American habit of making stomach a garbage disposal," "Diet fads are for the birds, if you don't like birds."

Hoffman, W. Meet Monsieur Cholesterol. University of Minnesota update, Winter, 1979, www.mbbnet.umn.edu/hoff/hoff_ak.html — In this interview Keys relates the anecdote about the man with knobs of cholesterol over his eyes.

Carroll. K. Experimental Evidence of Dietary Factors and Hormone-dependent Cancers. *Cancer Research* 35 (November 1975): 3374-3383. Data on tumorigenesis and caloric restriction, table 1, pg. 3375. Table 3, tumor rates as result of dietary restriction in mice, Table 1 and 2, p.3375 and 3376; ten-fold differences in cancer incidence rates between countries eating 50g fat/day as opposed to 140 g/day, p. 3578; cancer incidence as function of animal, vegetable and total fat, Table 3 and 4, p. 3379; breast cancer mortality strong correlation with animal protein intake, p. 3378; doubtful 5-10 fold differences explained by dietary intake of saturated fats alone, p. 3379.

Smith, Russell L. *Diet, Blood Cholesterol and Coronary Heart Disease: A Critical Review of the Literature.* 1991. Sherman Oaks, CA: Vector Enterprises. P. 4-47 to 4-49. High powered scientific sniping and rejection of Seven Countries Study.

Colditz, G., and S. Hankinson. The Nurses' Health Study: Lifestyle and Health among Women. *Nature Reviews/Cancer* 5 (May 2005): 388-396. Body mass and exercise studies, p. 393; $14/yr/participant, p. 394; 122,000 participants in 1976, 116,686 in 1989, p. 390; 90% follow up, 389; high vegetable fat intake related to low breast cancer incidence, high animal fat intake related to high colon cancer incidence, p.392; similar rates of breast cancer in high fat and low fat diets, Box 2, p. 392.

Hunter, D., D. Spiegelman, et al. Cohort Studies of Fat Intake and the Risk of Breast Cancer—A Pooled Analysis. *The New England Journal of Medicine* 334, no. 6 (February 1996): 356-361. "exponentiated the appropriate..." p. 357; "in the context of the western lifestyle..." p. 356; "no evidence..." p. 356; five-fold international breast cancer rates, descendants of migrants pick up incidence rates of new country; p.356.

Sun, Q., J. Ma, H. Campos, S. Hankinson, et al. A Prospective Study of Trans Fatty Acids in Erythrocytes and Risk of Coronary Heart Disease. *Circulation, Journal of the American Heart Association* 115 (2007): 1858-1865. Baseline trans fatty acid content in erythrocytes, study group:1.78% ± .44, control group: 1.66 ± .43%, Table 2, p.1860; 0.25% increase in trans fats linked to 30% increased coronary risk, p. 1861.

THE QUADRUPLE WHAMMY

Campbell, T. Colin, and Thomas M. Campbell III. 2006. *The China Study.* Dallas: Benbella Books. 27 years of research , p. 6; nearly 14% of GDP spent on health care, p. 18; every rat fed 20% protein got liver cancer or precursor lesions, no rat on 5% protein diet got cancer, p. 27; difference between correlation and causation in reductive scientific method, p. 39; "various factors," p. 47; eight essential amino acids, p. 30;

initiation, promotion, and metastasis of cancer, p. 49; chemical effects of protein on cancer, p. 53; cancer reawakened by bad nutrition later, p. 57; 100 week experiment of effect of casein on mice in which all the protein deprived mice lived and none of the control mice lived, p, 61; cancer rates 100 times or 10,000 percent different between regions, p. 71; American rates of heart disease and breast cancer 17 and 5 times higher than in parts of China, p. 79; average consumption of 35-40% calories as fat, p. 82; lack of fiber related to constipation type diseases, p. 89; Chart 5.3, heart disease mortality rates versus animal protein intake, p. 120; dietary changes reverse adverse coronary conditions, p. 130; "dairy intake is one of most consistent predictors..." p. 178; carnivorous nurses, p. 273-274; doctors receive 21 classroom hours of nutrition training in 4 years of medical school, p. 327; supercharged Vitamin D about 1000 times more active than Storage D, p. 362.

SORRY GUYS...SIZE MATTERS

Pollan, Michael. 2006. *The Omnivore's Dilemma.* New York: Penguin Books. Omega-6 inflammatory, omega-3 anti-inflammatory, p 268; grass finished beef has omega 6 to omega 3 ratio of 2:1, corn fed beef more than 10:1, p. 269.

en.wikipedia.org/wiki/Omega-3_fatty_acid#cite_note-85. — Section on omega-6 to omega-3 ratios good source of ratios in typical foods.

www.nal.usda.gov/fnic/foodcomp/search — This is the USDA website with a search engine for a detailed analysis of a large variety of processed and raw foods, and was used for the generalized protein/fat comparison of a 2000 calorie diet.

lipidlibrary.aocs.org/market/palmoil.htm — Palm oil processing.

MOLECULAR MIRACLES

Walker, Richard, ed. 2002. *Encyclopedia of the Human Body.* New York: Dorling Kindersley Limited.

Parker, Steve. 2007. *The Human Body Book.* New York: Dorling Kindersley Limited. Hydrophobic and hydrophilic phospholipids, p. 27.

lipidlibrary.aocs.org/index.html — Complex glycerolipids with detailed information on the structure and biologic function of all the important phospholipids, including phosphatidylcholine as diagrammed.

en.wikipedia.org/wiki/Linseed_oil — Fatty acid composition of flax oil.

Wang, L., J. Chen, and L. Thompson. The inhibitory effect of flaxseed on the growth and metastasis of estrogen receptor negative human breast cancer xenografts is attributed to both its lignan and oil components. *International Journal of Cancer* 116 (2005): 793-798. Flaxseed has lignin precursor levels 75-800 times that of other plants, p. 793; lignins shown to reduce metastasis, cell adhesion, migration, and invasion in vitro, dietary supplementation of 5-10% flax seed inhibits mammary cancer in mice, omega-3 fatty acids inhibit various stages of mammary carcinogenesis, p. 793; results of flax oil/lignin on breast cancer in mice study, p. 795-796; 10% flaxseed diet down-regulates 3 growth factors, including VEGF, IGF-1, EGFR, p. 796; enhancement of lipid peroxidation by n-3 fatty acids inhibits tumor growth, p. 196; in combination, lignins an oil complemented each other and triggered greater inhibitory effect, p. 797.

Thompson, L. U., J. M. Chen, T. Li, K. Strasser-Weippl, and P. Gross. Dietary Flaxseed Alters Tumor Biological Markers in Post-menopausal Breast Cancer. *Clinical Cancer Research* 11, no. 10 (May 2005): 3828-3835. Flax oil 57% omega-3, p. 3828; lignins both antioxidant and antiangiogenic, 100 to 800 times higher levels than 66 other typical plant foods, p. 3828; flaxseed affects initiation, growth and metastasis of mammary tumors in laboratory mice, p. 3829; 25 grams ground flaxseed per muffin, p. 3830; apotosis increased 30.7%, tumor cell proliferation decreased 34.2%, c-erB2 expression decreased 71% in flax groups as compared to control groups; 5-10% flaxseed diet in mice approximately equivalent to 25 g muffins in people, p. 3832; antiangiogenic effects of flaxseed supported by numerous preclinical studies, p. 3833.

THE BUDWIG PROTOCOL

rescomp.stanford.edu/~cheshire/EinsteinQuotes.html — Einstein quote.

Budwig, Johanna. 1992. *Flax Oil as a True Aid Against Arthritis, Heart Infarction, Cancer, and Other Diseases*, 3rd Ed. Vancouver: Apple Publishing Company, Limited, p. 1-59. Thread analogy, p. 7; unsaturated fatty acid chains easily form bonds with proteins, p. 7; "thus causing a recharging," p. 8; "enzymes of the breath can not function," p. 8; detrimental effects of trans fats increase with increasing number of trans bonds, p. 9; lack of highly unsaturated fats particularly noticeable with brain/nerve malfunctions, p. 12; di-polarity of fat/protein electric field crucially important, p. 17; flatly declare conventional cancer treatments cause cancer, p. 19; when you grind flax seed the triple unsaturated fatty acids break down in fifteen minutes, p. 22; "blue pigs" and "not suitable," p. 29; seven-time Nobel nominee, back cover.

Budwig, Johanna. 1994. *The Oil-Protein Diet Cookbook.* Vancouver: Apple Publishing Company, Limited, p. 1-178. Diets for the unwell and well alike.

Budwig, Johanna. Interview with Lothar Hirneise, excerpt from Budwig's 2005 book *Cancer—The Problem and the Solution.* Most easily accessible as reprint at: www.healingcancernaturally.com/lothar-hirneise -johanna-budwig.html — Senior expert for fats, p. 1; developed paper chromatography, p. 1; animals made asphyctic on diet of bleached rice, p. 2; "We cannot achieve something good with bad tools," about aversion to chemo and radiation, p. 5; attraction of fat to form lipoprotein increases as number of double bonds increases, stronger bond when you pull with both arms than one, triple bond as strong as a magnet, p. 5; quality of flaxseed varies greatly, p. 6; "if a woman has a very poor marriage...", p. 6; no one treatment right for everybody, p. 7; never claim to cure tumor with flax oil diet but there are examples..., p. 10.

ELECTRONS

Greene, Brian. 2000. *The Elegant Universe.* New York: Vintage Books. Newton says you can catch a beam of light, Einstein says no, p. 5; all force has associated particles, p. 11; individuals who are moving in respect to each other will not agree on their observations of time or space, p. 25; electromagnetic radiation 186,000 miles per second, p. 27; motion's effect on space and time, p. 47; electromagnetic wavelength and frequency, p. 89; Max Planck declared when it comes to energy, no fractions are allowed, thus ushering in the age of quantum mechanics, p. 92; double-slit experiments, p. 98-103; all matter has a wave like character, p. 104; electron location probability based on wavelength, p. 106; Feynman says electrons take every available path, p. 110; all measurements subject to error equal to wavelength of what is being measured, p. 111.

Bryson, Bill. 2003. *A Short History of Nearly Everything.* New York: Broadway Books. Human body equivalent to 30 large hydrogen bombs,

p. 122; a readable summation of particle physics over the last couple hundred years, p. 113-173.

Hawking, Stephen. 1996. *A Brief History of Time.* New York: Bantam Books. Orbits of electrons are functions of wavelengths that don't cancel each other out, p. 62; on the scale of atoms and molecules electromagnetic forces dominate, p. 73.

QIGONG

Holland, Alex. 1997. *Voices of Qi.* Berkeley: North Atlantic Books. Matter is condensed Qi, p. 1; other topics referenced more fully in chapter called "Yin, Yang and You."

The description of Qigong is from my own experience, augmented for accuracy from audiotapes recorded by Professor Hui Xian, next generation lineage holder for Turtle Longevity Qigong. More info: www.turtlelongevityqigong.org/index.htm.

EXTERNAL QI

Chen, K. W. An Analytic Review of Studies on Measuring Effects of External Qi in China. *Alternative Therapies* 10, no. 4 (July/August 2004): 38-50. Early experiments described in section on Physical Signal Detectors, p. 40-42; Paralyzed pig study, p. 45; increased oxidation rates, p. 42; affects on E-coli, p. 43.

Chen, Kevin, and Raphael Yeung. Exploratory Studies of Qigong Therapy for Cancer in China. *Integrative Cancer Therapies* 1, no. 4 (2002): 345-370. In Vitro Studies of EQ for cancer, Table 5, p. 355-357: relative size of cervical cells, Xu and Xin, 1992; qigong in addition to conventional radiation, Cao et al, 1993; Chen, et al, 1996, measured DNA synthesis, growth, metastasis factor in EQ versus sham treatments. Reviews of Clinical Studies of Qigong Therapy for cancer patients, Table 1, p. 348-351: comparing Qi, Chinese herbs and conventional chemotherapy, Fu et al, 1996; Stage III and IV patients show increased immune function and decreased side effects, Sun and Zhao, 1988. Reviews of In vivo studies of EQ therapy for cancer in animals: able 6, p. 360-363; tumor volume of EQ exposed cells less than half of control, Quian, et al, 1993.

Sancier, Kevin. Medical Applications of Qigong and Emitted Qi on Humans, Animals, Cell Cultures, and Plants: Review of Selected Scientific Research. *American Journal of Acupuncture* 19, no. 4 (1991): 367-377. Cultured sperm cell destroying/peaceful mind Qi, Table 3, p. 373; in vitro applied Qi increased natural killer cell indicators 20-50%, Table 4, p. 375.

Eisenberg, David, M.D. 1985. *Encounters With Qi.* New York: W.W. Norton and Company. Comrade Lin moving dart feather, p. 146-148.

TOO MANY OHMS IN THE MERIDIAN

Holland, Alex. 1997. *Voices of Qi.* Berkeley: North Atlantic Books.

Eisenberg, David, M.D. 1985. *Encounters With Qi.* New York: W.W. Norton and Company. Qi as anesthetic for brain surgery, p. 69-74.

Lo, Shui-Yin. Evidence and Mechanism of External Qi in Chinese Medicine. *Medical Acupuncture* 19, no. 4 (2007): 201-209. Skin temperature variation in response to EQ, Tables 1-5, p. 202-203.

Lo, Shui-Yin. Meridians in Acupuncture and Infra-red Imaging. *Medical Hypotheses* 58, no. 1 (2002): 72-76. Meridians composed of stable water clusters with permanent di-pole moment, p. 72.

YIN, YANG, AND YOU

Holland, Alex. 1997. *Voices of Qi.* Berkeley: North Atlantic Books. Microcosm reflects macrocosm, p. 2; yin and yang control, create, transform each other, p. 12; aspects of Yin and Yang, Table 1, p. 13; eight principles, p. 14-15; The five elements, Table 2, p. 16; mutual production cycle, Fig. 2, p. 16; pre- and post-natal Qi, p. 23; Chinese organ systems, p. 27-32; meridians, p. 32-38; dead fish story, p. 42.

Eisenberg, David, M.D. 1985. *Encounters With Qi.* New York: W.W. Norton and Company. Showcases full of hundreds of models of tongues, p. 52; six pulses in each wrist, p. 53; "Do you have the Qi?", p. 72; herbal medicine, p. 129.

MY HALF-LIFE AS A DIRTY BOMB

Burnett, N. G., R. Wurm, J. Nyman, and J. H. Peacock. Normal tissue sensitivity: How important is it? *Clinical Oncology* 8, no. 1 (1996): 25-34. 80% tissue variation in response to radiotherapy, p, 25.

Alsebeih, G., M. El-Sebaie, N. Al-Rajhi, A. Allam, M. Al-Buhairi, N. Al-Harbi, Y. Khafaga, M. Alsubael, and M. Al-Shabanah. Relationship between radiosensitivity and normal tissue, complications in Saudi cancer patients treated with radiotherapy. *Journal of the Egyptian Nat. Cancer Inst.* 16, no. 4 (2004): 216-233. Analysis of fibroblasts from 41 patients showed 3.5 fold differences in cell radiosensitivity, p. 220.

Prasad, K. Rationale for using multiple antioxidants in protecting humans against low doses of ionizing radiation. *The British Journal of Radiology* 78 (2005): 485-492. Radiation induced human cancers have latency periods of 10-30 years, p. 486; dependent on many factors, including DNA repair ability, p. 487; Vitamin E, A, Beta Carotene all protect normal tissue against radiation damage, p. 488; "it is possible..." p. 488.

Bolus, Norman. Basic Review of Radiation Biology and Terminology. *Journal of Nuclear Medical Technology* 29 (2001): 67-73. Interaction of radiation with cells is probability function, p. 67; energy deposition 10^{-18} second, p, 67; direct and indirect hits, p. 68; any radiation dose, no matter how small, can damage, p. 69; LD $_{50/30}$ in various species, Table 3, p. 70; Bergonie and Tribondeau, p. 67.

www.mdphysics.com/ncrp-report-no-160 — Data on increased population risk due to increased medical radiation.

en.wikipedia.org/wiki/Radioresistant — Radioresistance of various species.

en.wikipedia.org/wiki/Deinococcus_radiodurans — Conan the bacterium.

Grimm, P., J. Blasko, and J. Sylvester. 2003. *The Prostate Cancer Treatment Book*. New York: McGraw-Hill.

Lodish, H., A. Berk, P. Matsudaira, C. A. Kaiser, M. Krieger, M. P. Scott, S. L. Zipursky, and J. Darnell. 2004. *Molecular Biology of the Cell*, 5th Ed. New York: WH Freeman.

Berrington de Gonzalez, A., and S. Darby. Risk of cancer from diagnostic X-rays: estimates for the UK and 14 other countries. *The Lancet* 363 (January 31, 2004): 345-51. Increased risk of cancer due to diagnostic procedures increases with amount of procedures, 3.2% in Japan, 1.5% in Germany, 0.9% in US, Table 6, p. 349; weight of evidence there is no safe lower threshold below which radiation does not cause cancer. www.nytimes.com/2007/06/19/health/19cons.html?_r=1&n=Top%2f News%2fHealth%2fColumns%2fThe%20Consumer — Rise in medical radiation, from report issued by National Council on Radiation Protection and Measurements, Report 160.

IONIZING RADIATION

Shirazi, A., G. Ghobadi, and M. Ghazi-Khansari. A Radiobiological Review on Melatonin: A Novel Radioprotector. *Journal of Radiation Research* 48, no. 4 (2007): 263-272. Overview of free radical effect on DNA and speed of reaction, p. 264.

Umegaki, K., S. Ikegami, K. Inoue, T. Ichikawa, S. Kobayashi, N. Soeno, and K. Tomabechi. Beta Carotene prevents x-ray induction of micronuclei in human lymphocytes. *American Journal of Clinical Nutrition* 59 (1994): 409-412. Beta carotene as radioprotector.

en.wikipedia.org/wiki/DNA_repair — Molecular DNA lesions occur at rate of 1,000 to 1,000,000 per cell per day, numbers vary wildly because people vary wildly.

Terris, D., E. Ho, H. Ibrahim, M. Dorie, M. Kovacs, Q. Le, A. Koong, H. Pinto, and J. Brown. Estimating DNA Repair by Sequential Evaluation of Head and Neck Tumor Radiation Sensitivity Using the Comet Assay. *Arch Otolaryngol Head Neck Surgery* 128 (2002): 698-702. DNA repair rates in cancer cells, half-life of 4.2 minutes, p. 698; ionizing radiation induces 3-4 times fewer DNA breaks in anaerobic than aerobic cells, p. 699; 15 Gray damage repaired in 30 minutes to 2 hours, p. 699; "There appears to be no significant difference in the DNA repair rate between tumor and normal cells," p. 699; solid tumors are known to be heterogeneous, p. 700; hypoxia marker for radiation resistance and tumor aggressiveness, p. 700.

Peehl, D. Primary cell cultures as models of prostate cancer development. *Endocrine-Related Cancer* 12 (2005): 19-47. 15-LOX-2, involved in arachidonic acid metabolism, reduced in matched cancer culture, virtually absent in established cancer cell lines, p. 31; flavinoid, allyl isothyiocyanate (in cruciferous vegetables), Vitamin D, retinoids, lycopene all helped kill cancer cells while not harming normal cells in vitro, p. 34-35; "Given that radiotherapy is a widely used treatment option...", p. 37; cancer attributable to alterations in phospholipids membrane, p. 38.

Bromfield, G. P., A. Meng, P. Warde, and R. G. Bristow. Cell death in irradiated prostate epithelial cells: role of apoptotic and clonogenic cell kill. *Prostate Cancer and Prostatic Diseases* 6 (2003): 73-85. "Suggesting that malignant cells are more radioresistant than normal prostate cells, for this series," p. 73; results, Figure 2, p. 78.

Dunlap, N., G. G. Schwartz, D. Eads, S. D. Cramer, A. B. Sherk, V. John, and C. Koumenis. 1α,25,Dihydroxyvitamin D3 (Calcitriol) and its analogue, 19-nor-1 α,25$(OH)_2D_2$, potentiate the effects of ionizing radiation on human prostate cancer cells. *British Journal of Cancer* 89 (2003): 746-753. Higher radiation doses lead to more morbidity, especially rectal bleeding, p. 746; greater synergism at IR of 2gy, p. 751; tenfold decrease in radiation with supplemental Vitamin D to achieve same effect, p. 751.

Girdhani. S., S. M. Bhosle, S. A. Thulsidas, A. Kumar, and K. P. Mishra. Potential of radiosensitizing agents in cancer chemo-radiotherapy. *Journal of Cancer Research Therapy* 1, no. 3 (September 2005). Cancer cells are deficient in poly-unsaturated fatty acids rendering them chemo- and radio-resistant, p. 129; Vitamin E induces apoptosis in cancer cells most likely by changing plasma membrane fluidity, 130; triphala made cancer cells less resistant to radiation while sparing normal cells.

THE WARBURG EFFECT

Gillispie, Charles Coulston, ed. 1976. *Dictionary of Scientific Biography*, Volume XIV. New York: Charles Scribner's Sons, p. 1-640. Max Planck quote, p. 173; "oxygen dethroned" and "prime cause," p. 176; medieval lance, p. 173; B-vitamins as a cure for cancer, p. 176; discovered lactic acid/tumor connection, p. 176.

Warburg, Otto. The Prime Cause and Prevention of Cancer, presented at 1966 meeting of Nobel laureates. English translation by Dan Burk, National Cancer Institute, a copy can be found at www.hopeforcancer.com/OxyPlus.htm. "Cancer, above all other diseases..." p. 1; mice sicken with tetanus shows low oxygen, p. 1; mouse embryos develop cancer when oxygen pressures drop to 65% of normal, p. 3; "During the development of cancer the oxygen-respiration always fails...", p. 5, "prophets of agnosticism..." p. 7.

Hammarsten, E. Nobel Prize for Physiology in 1931, presentation speech, at nobelprize.org/nobel_prizes/medicine/laureates/1931/press.html — "rare perfection in the art of measurement."

Warburg, O., F. Wind, and E. Negelein. The Metabolism of Tumors in the Body. *The Journal of General Physiology* (March 1927): 519-530. Chicken and forearm experiments, p. 519; 46 milligrams of lactic acid increase, p. 525; glucose changes in normal tissue versus tumor, p. 522; died in about four hours, p. 521; "resistance of a single tumor is not to be compared...", p. 521; "only a thin outer layer..." in experiment on rats in low oxygen, p. 529; "At first it seems paradoxical...", p. 530.

en.wikipedia.org/wiki/Otto_Heinrich_Warburg — eccentric nature.

HYPOXIA

Dewhirst, M. W., Y. Cao, and B. Moeller. Cycling hypoxia and free radicals regulate angiogenesis and radiotherapy response. *Nature Reviews/Cancer* 8 (June 2008): 425-437. Drop to 10 mm oxygen induces HIF-1, p. 425; effects of HIF-1, p. 425; presence of hypoxia well established source of resistance to radiation therapy and chemotherapy, p. 428; intermittent hypoxia cause for radioresistance, p. 429; two waves of hypoxia, p. 429; cycling hypoxia increase free radical levels, p. 431; stress granules, p. 534.

Marignol, L., M. Coffey, M. Lawler, and D. Hollywood. Hypoxia in prostate cancer: A powerful shield against tumour destruction? *Cancer Treatment Reviews* 34 (2008): 313-327. Tumor hypoxia intimately associated with tumor progression, p. 315; hypoxia affects treatment resistance and apoptosis, p. 316; multi-drug resistance protein, p. 319; hypoxic cells commonly three times more radioresistant than normoxic cells, p. 320; hypoxia a factor that triggers adaptation and treatment resistance in cancer, p. 321.

Dang, C., J. Kim, P. Gao, and J. Yustein. The Interplay between MYC and HIF in cancer. *Nature Reviews/Cancer* 8, no. 1 (January 2008): 51-56. Three separate HIF proteins, p. 51; free radicals stabilize HIF levels and actively suppress respiration, p. 52; antioxidants dramatically suppress tumorigenesis, p. 53; hypoxic tissues if greater than 100 microns from oxygen source, p. 54; dramatic increase in glucose uptake by tumors, p. 54.

en.wikipedia.org/wiki/HIF-1 — HIF-1 highly conserved in oxygen-breathers.

plato.stanford.edu/entries/aristotle-logic — One of many sources for information on Aristotelian logic and syllogisms.

Harrison, L., M. Chadha, R. Hill, K. Hu, and D. Shasha. Impact of Tumor Hypoxia and Anemia on Radiation Therapy Outcomes. *The Oncologist* 7 (2002): 492-508. Anemia common in cancer population and contributes to hypoxia, p. 492-493; during radiotherapy risk of anemia increases 80%, p. 493; tumors are heterogeneous, p. 493; intratumoral oxygen level most significant factor in radiotherapy effectiveness, p. 494, p. 502; hypoxia increases during radiation and chemotherapy, p. 494.

National Institutes of Health, Office of Dietary Supplements, Dietary Supplement Fact Sheet: Iron. dietary-supplements.info.nih.gov/factsheets/iron.asp — Check out this NIH website for very good information on anemia and how to remedy it.

Tonelli, M., B. Hemmelgarn, T. Reiman, B. Manns, M. Reaume, A. Lloyd, N. Wiebe, and S. Klarenbach. Benefits and harms of erythropoiesis-stimulating agents for anemia related to cancer: a meta-analysis. *Canadian Medical Association Journal* (May 26, 2009). 16% increased risk of death due to antianemia drugs, p. E68.

Zajusz, A., B. Maciejewski, et al. Normobaric oxygen as a sensitizer in radiotherapy for advanced head and neck cancer. *Neoplasma* 42, no. 3 (1995): 137-40. Three year survival 19% in treated group, 2% in control, p. 137.

Haffty, B. G., R. Hurley, and L. J. Peters. Radiation therapy with hyperbaric oxygen at 4 atmospheres in the management of squamous cell carcinoma of the head and neck: results of a randomized clinical trial. *Cancer J Sci Am* 5, no. 6 (November/December 1999): 334-5. No significant differences in metastasis or 5 yr. survival, p. 335.

Block, K. Antioxidants and Cancer Therapy: Furthering the Debate. *Integrative Cancer Therapies* 3, no. 4 (2004): 342-348. Heated debate on whether to use antioxidants with radiation and/or chemotherapy, p. 342.

Kumar, B., M. Jha, W. Cole, J. Bedford, and K. Prasad. D-Alpha-Tocopheryl Succininate (Vitamin E) Enhances Radiation-Induced Chromosomal Damage Levels in Human Cancer Cells, but Reduces it in Normal Cells. *Journal of the American College of Nutrition* 21, no. 4 (2002): 339-343. Vitamin E enhanced radiation induce chromosomal damage in cancer cells, protected normal cells from damage, p. 339; Vitamin C and A have similar effects in vitro and in vivo, p. 341; results, Fig. 1, p. 341.

Lee, T., R. Johnke, R. Allison, K. O'Brien, and L. Dobbs. Radioprotective potential of ginseng. *Mutagenesis* 20, no. 4 (2005): 237-243. Whole plant better than isolated fractions, effective as radioprotector p. 237; over 200 chemicals, p. 238; ginsenosides associated with antioxidant, antistress, antidiabetic, antineoplastic, and have proved beneficial in cardiovascular, endocrine, immune, and central nervous systems, p. 238.

Shirazi, A., G. Ghobadi, M. Ghazi-Khansari. A Radiological Review on Melatonin: A Novel Radioprotector. *Journal Radiation Research* 48, no. 4 (2007): 263-272. Half-life of free radicals 10^{-6} to 10^{-10} seconds, p. 264; 60-70% of radiation damage caused by free radicals, p. 264; melatonin synthesized by pineal gland, p. 266; melatonin at physiological doses induces apoptosis in cancer cells, lowers metastatic tendencies, reduces tumor growth in variety of in vivo and in vitro experiments, p. 268; acts as an antioxidant in lipids and proteins (glutathione), wide ranging antioxidant and radioprotecting attributes, p. 266-267.

www.lef.org/protocols/cancer/radiation_therapy_01.htm — A good overview with references to improving radiotherapy outcomes with complementary medicine.

THERE'S A TUMOR IN MY SWEET TOOTH

Walker, Richard, ed. 2002. *Encyclopedia of the Human Body.* New York: Dorling Kindersley Limited. Typically 5 g glucose in 5 liters human blood, p. 200; respiration, p.23.

Parker, Steve. 2007. *The Human Body Book.* New York: Dorling Kindersley Limited.

Blood sugar regulation, p. 110, diabetes, p. 111.

diabetes.niddk.nih.gov/dm/pubs/overview — One measure of diabetes is 200 mg/dl of glucose in non-fasting blood.

www.acaloriecounter.com/candy-chocolate.php — Grams of glucose in popular candies, there is also a quick link to grams of glucose in popular cereals.

Griggs, B. 1997. *Green Pharmacy: The History and Evolution of Western Herbal Medicine.* Rochester, Vermont: Healing Arts Press. 60,000-year-old medicinal plants, p. 1.

Ghururaj, A. E., M. Belakavadi, et al. Molecular mechanisms of anti-angiogenic effect of curcumin. *Biochem Biophys Res Commun* 297, no. 4 (October 4, 2002): 934-42. Curcumin induced apoptosis and inhibited angiogenesis in vivo, p. 934.

Yang, S., N. Lin, et al. Anti-angiogenic effect of silymarin on colon cancer LoVo cell line. *J Surg Res* 113, no. 1 (July 2003): 133-8. Silymarin significantly inhibits in vitro cancer cell growth and angiogenesis, p. 137; nontoxic in acute doses, p. 133.

Seidlova-Wuttke, D., T. Becker, V. Christoffel, H. Jarry, and W. Wuttke. Silymarin is a selective estrogen receptor B (ERB) agonist and has estrogenic effects in the metaphysics of the femur but no or antiestrogenic effects in the uterus of ovariectomized (ovx) rats. *Journal of Steroid Biochemistry and Molecular Biology* 86, no. 2 (2003): 179-188. Silybinin, major component of silymarin, binds to estrogen receptors, p. 179.

Fowke, J., J. Morrow, S. Motley, R. Bostick, and R. Ness. Brassica vegetable consumption reduces urinary F2-isoprostane levels independent of micronutrient intake. *Carcinogenesis* 27, no. 10 (2006): 2096-2102. Vegetable burgers don't cure cancer, p. 2096; F2-isoprostane gold standard measure of lipid peroxidation, p. 2097; urinary levels of F2-iso increased about 22% above control, p. 2098.

Xiao, et al. Allyl isothiocyanate, a constituent of cruciferous vegetables, inhibits proliferation of human prostate cancer cells by causing G2/M arrest and inducing apoptosis. *Carcinogenesis* 24 (2003): 891-897. Significantly increased apoptosis due to allyl isothiocyanate in cultured cancer cells, p. 891.

Heggie, S., G. Bryant, L. Tripcony, J. Keller, P. Rose, M. Glendenning, and J. Heath. A Phase III Study on the Efficacy of Topical Aloe Vera Gel on Irradiated Breast Tissue. *Cancer Nursing* 25, no. 6 (December 2002): 442-451. Study showing aloe did not significantly improve radiation burn.

Olsen, D. L., W. Raub, Jr., et al. The effect of aloe vera gel mild soap versus mild soap alone in preventing skin reactions in patients undergoing radiation therapy. Oncol Nurs Forum 28, no. 3 (2001): 543-547. Just to be fair, another study showing aloe did significantly improve radiation burn.

REEFER MADNESS

Earlywine, M. 2002. *Understanding Marijuana, A New Look at the Scientific Evidence.* New York: Oxford University Press. Anandamide, p. 139; fruit flies to molluscs, p. 138; more than 60 compounds plus complex nature of cannabinoid interaction, p. 120-124; hemp fibers, early uses, rope p. 4; first medical use, p. 10; cannabis, ephedra, and Emperor Shen Neng; p. 10; hemp for victory, p. 6; prescribed for diverse ailments,

p. cost of dronanbinol, p. 16; sperm count and motility, p. 159; Indian bhang drinkers; anti-emetic properties 1975 New England Journal of Medicine study, p. 180; increased appetite, p. 182; 5% weight loss detrimental, p. 183; 50%-80% of cancer patients show cachexia or wasting; dronabinol cost, p. 170; number of marijuana smokers worldwide and in America, p. 29-30, low addictive qualities, p. 32; Jamaican men smoking 20 joints a day, p. 79; can't remember beginning of sentence, p. 110; CB1 and CB2 receptors, p. 136-137.

De Petrocellis, L., D. Melck, T. Bisogno, A. Milone, and V. De Marzo. Finding of the endocannabinoid signaling system in Hydra, a very primitive organism: possible role in the feeding response. *Neuroscience* 92, no.1 (1999): 377-387. Retrograde feeding response and existence of cannabinoid receptors in hydra, p. 377.

en.wikipedia.org/wiki/Hydra_(genus) — Hydra biology.

From British parliament on the history of cannabis: www.parliament .the-stationery-office.co.uk/pa/ld199798/ldselect/ldsctech/151/ 15103.htm — "consumeth the wind and drieth the seed," from 1597 Herbal by botanist John Gerard.

Pride, E. The Endocannabinoid-CB Receptor System: Importance for development and in pediatric disease. *Neuroendocrinology Letters* 25, no. 1/2 (February/April 2004): 24-30. CB arrest development of 2 cell mouse embryos, p. 25; development of suckling response, p. 26-27; neural development, p. 24.

dailymed.nlm.nih.gov/dailymed/archives/fdaDrugInfo.cfm?archive id=16800 — NIH drug info website; the artificial cannabinoid pharmaceutical described is nabilone, with a chemical formula of $C_{24}H_{36}O_3$, while THC is $C_{21}H_{30}O_2$; dog and monkey trial under "animal pharmacology" heading; "virtually all the patients who received this drug experienced at least one adverse reaction," under heading of "adverse reactions."

Guzman, M. Cannabinoids: Potential Anticancer Agents. *Nature Reviews/Cancer* 3 (October 2003): 743-755. CB1 and CB2 expression, p. 745; anti-emitic qualities at least equivalent to typical pharmaceuticals, p. 746; retrograde signaling pathway, p. 747; cachexia and 5% weight loss, p. 747, cannabinoids inhibit pain, p. 748; nine kinds of cancer affected by four signaling pathways, Table 2, p. 749; inhibit tumor growth, metastasis, angiogenesis and induce apotosis, p. 750.

Solowji, N., R. Stephens, R. Roffman, et al. Cognitive Functioning of Long-Term Heavy Cannabis Users Seeking Treatment. *Journal of the American Medical Association* 287, no. 9 (2002): 1123-1131. An ounce a month for 24 years study; past research clearly demonstrates gross impairment not related to chronic cannabis use, p. 1123; comparison of cognitive effects, Table 3, p. 1127.

Leape, L. Scope of Problem and History of Patient Safety. *Obstetrics and Gynecology Clinics of North America* 35 (2008): 1-10. Adverse pharmaceutical reactions, p. 1.

Papathanasopoulos, P., L. Messinis, E. Lyros, A. Kastellakis, and G. Panagis. Multiple Sclerosis, Cannabinoids, and Cognition. *Journal of Neuropsychiatry and Clinical Neurosciences* 20, no. 1 (Winter 2008): 36-51.

www.pfizer.com/files/products/uspi_xanax_xr.pdf.

THE KISS OF DEATH

Walker, Richard, ed. 2002. *Encyclopedia of the Human Body.* New York: Dorling Kindersley Limited. Acquired immune response pathway, p. 160-161; lymph and lymph nodes, p. 154-155, lymph-blood relationship, 3-4 liters a day pass through lymph system, p. 152; fist-sized spleen, p. 155.

Parker, Steve. 2007. *The Human Body Book.* New York: Dorling Kindersley Limited. Complement system of proteins, p. 159; lymph and lymph nodes, p. 158; macrophage, antigen, T-cell relationship, p. 153; viral attack, p. 162-163; B cells and T cells that hang out in the spleen and together manufacture acquired immunity, p. 159.

en.wikipedia.org/wiki/Major_histocompatibility_complex — A good overview of major histocompatibility complex.

Zamai, L., C. Ponti, P. Mirandola, G. Gobbi, S. Papa, L Galeotti, L. Gocco, and M. Vitale. NK Cells and Cancer. *The Journal of Immunology* 178 (2007): 4011-4016. Natural killer cells central role in control and identification of tumor growth and metastasis, p. 4011.

Cerwenka, A., and L. Lanier . Natural Killer Cells, Viruses, and Cancer. *Nature Reviews/Immunology* 1 (October, 2001): 41-49. Natural killers originally discovered because of ability to kill tumors, p. 41; many inhibitory and activating receptors/signals involved in tumor surveillance, Tables 1 and 2, p. 42-43; NK cells are regulated by a balance between activating and inhibitory signals, thus can kill tumors; p. 43; histological examination of tumors rarely finds NK cells, p. 47.

Block, K., and M. Mead. Immune System Effects of Echinacea, Ginseng, and Astragalus: A Review. *Integrative Cancer Therapies* 2, no. 3 (2003): 247-267. Prairie coneflower, p. 249; three species prepared in different ways yield huge variation in commercial products, p. 249-250; polysaccharides, cichoric acid and alkamides, p. 250; immune boosting chemicals in ginseng, p. 254, immune boosting in astragalus, p. 256, wide variation in commercial ginseng preparations, p. 254.

Miller, S. Echinacea: a Miracle Herb against Aging and Cancer? Evidence in vivo in Mice. *Evidence-based Complementary and Alternative Medicine* 2, no. 3 (2005): 309-314. Arabinogalactin, alkamide, cichoric acid, and related cytokines relationship, p. 310; Echinacea appears to be tailor made to stimulate innate immune system, p. 310; no *in vivo* toxic level, p. 310; Echinacea in mice pro-rated to humans, p. 311; young healthy mice, p. 310; old healthy mice, p. 311; prophylactic use, p. 312; whole plant preferable to isolated compounds, p. 312; cancerous mice, p. 313; melatonin is another powerful NK stimulant, p. 313; humans and mice are 97% genetically similar.

Currier, N. L., and S. E. Miller. Echinacea purpurea and melatonin augment natural killer cells in leukemic mice and prolong life span. *Journal of Alternative and Complementary Medicine* 7, no. 3 (2001): 241-251. 2-3 fold increase in NK cells at nine days and three months in leukemic mice receiving Echinacea in their chow, p. 241; 1/3 of both Echinacea and melatonin groups survived to three months and beyond, p. 245; increase in NK cells best natural defense against cancer, increase in NK cells does reflect increase in functional armament available, p. 247; no tumor cells found at three months, p. 248.

Independent nutrient analysis, Consumerlab.com.

Turner, R. B., et al. An Evaluation of Echinacea augustifolia in Experimental Rhinovirus Infections. *New England Journal of Medicine* 353 (2005): 341-8. No one preparation had high quantities of all three active ingredients; first preparation had 0% polysaccharides, 73.8% alkamides, second preparation had 48.9% polysaccharides, 2.3% alkamides; third had 42.1 polysaccharides, 0.11 % alkamides. No cichoric acid was found in any sample, and no echinocasides were found in any sample. P. 344.

Shah, S., S. Sander, C. White, M. Rinaldi, and C. Coleman. Evaluation of echinacea for the prevention and treatment of the common cold: a meta-analysis. *The Lancet Infectious Diseases* 7, no. 7 (July 2007): 473-480. Criticizes Turner study for using dose of 1 gram instead of recommended 3 grams, p. 479; 86% reduction in combination with Vitamin C, p. 478; 58% reduction, p. 473.

IT DOESN'T MATTER WHAT YOU BELIEVE, AS LONG AS YOU BELIEVE

Ader, R. Behaviorally Conditioned Immunosuppression. Letter to the Editor, *Psychosomatic Medicine* 36, no. 2 (March/April 1974): 183-84. Describing how pigs died in response to sweetened water, p. 183; "gastrointestinal distress," p. 183.

Bovbjerg, D. H., W. H. Redd, L. A. Maier, J. C. Holland, L. M. Lesko, D. Niedzwiecki, S. C. Rubin, and T. B. Hakes. Anticipatory immune suppression and nausea in women receiving cyclic chemotherapy for ovarian cancer. *Journal of Consulting and Clinical Psychology* 58, no. 2 (April 1990):153-7.

Price, D., D. Finniss, and F. Benedetti. A Comprehensive Review of the Placebo Effect: Recent Advances and Current Thought. *Annual Review of Psychology* 59 (2008): 565-90. Anise flavored syrup and MS patients, p 580; "The focus has shifted from the "inert" content...", p. 567; magnitude of placebo response 39%, 26.9%, and 56% in three different studies, p. 569; placebo effect varies from large to small and doesn't affect everybody, p. 569; open-hidden paradigm, p. 568; five commonly used pain relieving drugs experiment, Figure 1, p. 569; "conscious expectation is necessary...", p. 571; balloon barostat experiment, including quotations as to intent, p. 572; desire and expectation are multiplicative factors in placebo effect, p. 572; goal, focus, desire, expectation and mood affect placebo effect, p. 574-575; somatic focus (patients reported more placebo relief when they focused on symptoms), p. 575.

Segerstrom, S., and G. Miller. Psychological Stress and the Human Immune System: A Meta-Analytic Study of 30 Years of Inquiry. *Psychological Bulletin* 130, no. 4 (2004): 601-630. As humans age the immune system becomes senescent, p. 605; acute stress, mental math and public speaking, p. 607; brief stress, taking tests, p. 612; chronic stress, dementia caregiving, unemployment; p. 614; chemical and physical pathways between immune and nervous stress systems, p. 604; chronic stress depressed nearly every immune function, Table 7, p. 615.

Sephton, S., C. Koopman, M. Schall, C. Thoresen, and D. Spiegel. Spiritual Expression and Immune Status in Women with Metastatic Breast Cancer: An Exploratory Study. *The Breast Journal* 7, no. 5 (2002): 345-353. Women with breast cancer who reported greater spirituality had higher levels of helper and cytotoxic T cells, p. 345.

Broadbent, E., K. Petrie, C. Ellis, J. Ying, and G. Gamble. A picture of health-myocardial infarction patients & apos; drawings of their hearts and subsequent disability: A longitudinal study. *Journal of Psychosomatic Research* 57, no. 6 (2004): 583-587. 74 consecutive patients following admittance to a hospital for myocardial infarction drew pictures of how much damage they thought their hearts had sustained, the pictures better predicted recovery than standard blood tests, p. 583.

I FISH THEREFORE I AM

Bryson, B. 2004. *A Short History of Nearly Everything.* New York: Broadway Books, p. 1-544. Whatever prompted life to begin, it happened only once, p. 293; organic molecules on incoming comets, p. 292; life began 3.85 billion years ago, crust became solid 3.9 billion years ago, p. 292; inhospitable and volatile nature of Archean world, p. 297; arrival of oxygen, mitochondria and eukaryotes, p. 300; every day billions of cells commit apoptosis; p. 379; oceans formed 3.8 billion years ago, same water now, p. 272.

Leakey, R., and R. Lewin. 1995. *The Sixth Extinction: Patterns of Life and the Future of Mankind.* New York: Anchor Books, p. 1-271. Hardening of crust, p. 14; eukaryotes and prokaryotes, p. 15; Cambrian explosion and vertebrates, p. 17.

Whitman, W., D. Coleman, and W. Wiebe. Prokaryotes: The unseen majority. *Proceedings of the National Academy of Sciences* 95 (June 1998): 6578-6583. Ocean cell density, p. 6578, soil cell density, p. 6579; colon cell density, p. 6580.

www.pbs.org/wgbh/evolution/change/deeptime/protero.html — Concise info on the rise of atmospheric oxygen during Proterozoic time.

THE END OF THE BEGINNING

rex.nci.nih.gov/NCI_Pub_Interface/raterisk/rates24.html — Female breast cancer highest among white women in the San Francisco area (104.2), lowest among women in The Gambia (3.4 per 100,000). Prostate cancer rates highest for black men in Atlanta, Georgia (102.0), lowest in Qidong, China (0.8 per 100,000). 1992 data.

Hoffman, W. Meet Monsieur Cholesterol. University of Minnesota update, Winter, 1979, www.mbbnet.umn.edu/hoff/hoff_ak.html — "Diet fads..."

Vinson, Joe. University of Scranton, Polyphenols found in popcorn, snacks, and whole grain cereals, at the 238th annual national meeting of the American Chemical Society. www.ustream.tv/recorded/2004849) — This is the link to hear the talk.

law.justia.com/us/cfr/title21/21-2.0.1.1.23.2.1.11.html — This links to the code of federal regulations, Title 21, Part 37, 137.200...definition of whole wheat flour. If you want to know why you can't tell what's in your food, check it out.

www.ers.usda.gov/Data/BiotechCrops — USDA data on increasing amount of genetically altered corn, soybeans, cotton planted in U.S. from 1996-2010.

www.nature.com/horizon/proteinfolding/background/disease.html — Improperly folded proteins form insoluble plaques associated with Alzheimer's.

Index

About the Author

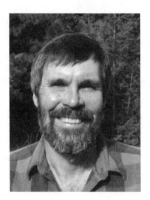

Dave Ames is the author of three books about fly fishing and one book about cancer. He prefers fishing to having cancer, so when he got diagnosed and heard the dire odds, he set about trying to prove the doctors wrong. Cancer-free for several years now, he's on a mission to tell others how he did it.

Dave grew up on the shores of Lake Erie. He was one of those kids who read Mark Twain and the Hardy Boys late into the night by a flashlight hidden under a blanket. Fishing came naturally to him. He graduated with a degree in geology from Allegheny College, and became a fly-fishing guide. He has spoken to audiences in the tens of thousands, in venues all over the country, and has kept his listeners roaring with laughter. He's been interviewed on regional and national television, and has written for a variety of newspapers and magazines.

Dave lives in Missoula, Montana, where he's been known to do a bit of fishing now and then.

Sentient Publications, LLC publishes books on cultural creativity, experimental education, transformative spirituality, holistic health, new science, ecology, and other topics, approached from an integral viewpoint. Our authors are intensely interested in exploring the nature of life from fresh perspectives, addressing life's great questions, and fostering the full expression of the human potential. Sentient Publications' books arise from the spirit of inquiry and the richness of the inherent dialogue between writer and reader.

Our Culture Tools series is designed to give social catalyzers and cultural entrepreneurs the essential information, technology, and inspiration to forge a sustainable, creative, and compassionate world.

We are very interested in hearing from our readers. To direct suggestions or comments to us, or to be added to our mailing list, please contact:

SENTIENT PUBLICATIONS, LLC
1113 Spruce Street
Boulder, CO 80302
303-443-2188
contact@sentientpublications.com
www.sentientpublications.com